VITAMIN D
VITAMIN C IODINE

Why more is better

Alexandre Doumenach MD

This book is not a medical textbook. This book cannot be a
substitute for a medical consultation. It is only a collection of
information on many diseases. Any suggestions contained in
the book are also information only. Any attempt to treat the
disease should be done in cooperation with the doctor. The
author is not responsible for the consequences of using the
information contained in the book for therapeutic purposes.

I dedicate this book to my wife and children because the thought of them drives me; Kazimiera and Gemma for supporting me spiritually; and all doctors who have dedicated their lives to seeking the truth.

CONTENTS

INTRODUCTION

I have known Dr. Alexandre Doumenach for over 40 years, since our medical school in Paris. It can therefore be said that I know him well and I have learned his character thoroughly. Already several dozen years ago, he impressed me a lot. He was very hardworking. He was one of the best students who whenever he had any doubts, after lectures he always tried to dispel them by asking professors. The search for truth has always been an integral part of his life. He also often helped others when they didn't understand or know something. Meetings where he taught other students were organized. This part of the character hasn't changed either. I am very grateful to be able to write an introduction to his book, which expresses his great personality and aims to convey the truth and help others, so that in the world we live in there may be less unnecessary suffering. This book also expresses something else - courage. Dr. Doumenach was not afraid to write a book that not everyone would like, especially pharmaceutical companies that spend billions on using their products and not some cheap vitamins or minerals. These natural substances would not bring such a profit to anyone and the patient could be cured forever. This is what this book is about; about three amazing substances that promote health.

Dr. Alexandre Doumenach shows, based on many scientific studies, that diseases and conditions such as cancer, atherosclerosis, heart attack, stroke, hypertension, diabetes (both type 1 and type 2), colds, COVID-19, pneumonia, sepsis, Parkinson's disease, Alzheimer's disease, multiple sclerosis, autism, asthma, psoriasis, eczema, acne, rheumatoid arthritis, polycystic ovary syndrome (PCOS), endometriosis, osteoporosis, infertility, migraines, depression, obesity, fibrocystic breast disease , thyroid disease (hypothyroidism, hyperthyroidism, autoimmune thyroiditis) and fibromyalgia can be significantly prevented, alleviated and even cured. He points out that we need more of these substances; vitamin D, vitamin C and iodine.

Therefore, the subtitle of this book is "why more is better." And it is true. Maybe the commonly recommended dose of vitamin C will prevent scurvy, maybe the commonly recommended dose of iodine will prevent goiter, but it certainly will not prevent the diseases and ailments mentioned above. This, referring to each subsequent scientific publication, reveals Dr. Doumenach. It should also be added that he perfectly chose the substances he will write about, i.e. vitamin D, vitamin C and iodine. These are substances with which a lot of solid studies have been conducted, many healthy and sick people are deficient in them, they are cheap, and most importantly, they are extremely effective in preventing and treating diseases.

Dr. Doumenach begins each chapter with a brief introduction, in which he often points to the mechanism of substances in a particular disease entity and prevalence of deficiency. Then he moves to the most important - scientific studies, which are plentiful. This is a feature that sets this book apart from others. The author usually gives details of these studies, including the number of subjects, the dose, and the exact results. Thanks to this, the reader can see a clear picture of the situation and the great abilities of the substance. Thanks to this, the book is also extremely credible. The book is not a collection of the author's beliefs but facts backed up by studies. Unfortunately, most of the books on similar topics are either not based on studies at all or only to a small extent, and most pages are filled with anecdotes and various stories. In the case of Dr. Alexandre Doumenach's book, it is completely different. In addition, the studies referred to in the book, apart from their large number, are also of various types, ranging from meta-analyzes, randomized controlled trials, cohort studies to case reports. It also gives a clearer picture, e.g. which doses of substances give better results.

Importantly, at the end of each section devoted to each element, the author draws conclusions about the safety and optimal dose for maintaining health. It turns out that all three substances are extremely safe. Higher levels of vitamin D than these recommended do not cause kidney calcification, vitamin C does not cause kidney stones, and iodine does not cause hyperthyroidism, among other things. Studies and experienced doctors, in turn, indicate that we should consume higher doses of these essential substances to stay healthy and recover quickly in case of illness.

Who is this book for? I think for everyone. For everyone who wants to prevent disease and live a healthy life as well as for everyone who is struggling with some disease now. It is very likely that the information in this book will help the person overcome this disease or at least alleviate the unwanted symptoms. Finally, this book is for any physician who wants to broaden their understanding of treatment and treat their own patients effectively. The number of scientific publications on which the book is based will undoubtedly help to achieve this.

- Bernard Fontaine MD

PART I: VITAMIN D

CHAPTER 1:
CANCER

Cancer is one of the most feared diseases. No wonder as it often leads to death. Even if luckily it doesn't happen to us, cancer has a devastating effect on both our body and our psyche, and may lead to anxiety or depression. Our relatives and friends also suffer then. Worse, the future is not very bright. In the United States, it is estimated that one in two women and one in three men will develop cancer in their lifetime. Similar estimates are also reported in other countries. Little is said about prevention, although there is much evidence that cancer risk can be significantly reduced. And vitamin D, vitamin C and iodine play a big role here. We will start with vitamin D, which has a strong anti-cancer effect, both in terms of prevention and treatment.

Laboratory and animal studies have shown that vitamin D has anti-inflammatory, immunomodulatory, antiangiogenic (reducing the unwanted growth of cancerous blood vessels) and proapoptotic (promoting death of cancer cells) properties. Vitamin D inhibits carcinogenesis and slows tumor progression. Vitamin D may also reduce mortality by reducing tumor invasiveness as well as propensity to metastasize. Higher levels of vitamin D (25(OH)D) have been associated by many studies with both a lower incidence of cancer and a higher survival rate of cancer patients. We will try to take a closer look at these studies and at the same time various types of cancers. This will give us a more accurate picture of which path we should choose as a society and at least what levels of vitamin D should be targeted to reduce the risk as much as possible.

Colorectal cancer

The first type of cancer we will deal with is colorectal cancer. Annually, around 2,000,000 new cases of this cancer are diagnosed worldwide. Statistics show that the lifetime risk of developing colorectal cancer is: about 1 in 23 for men and 1 in 25 for women. In addition, about a million people die from this ailment each year, which makes this cancer one of the most deadly. Hence, it is so important to determine whether it can be prevented and to what extent. We will discuss this on the basis of various pieces of evidence.

Grant, W.B., & Garland, C.F. (2006). **The association of solar ultraviolet B (UVB) with reducing risk of cancer: multifactorial ecologic analysis of geographic variation in age-adjusted cancer mortality rates**. Anticancer research, 26 4A, 2687-99 .

Dr. Grant and Dr. Garland analyzed the colon cancer mortality rates in different counties (1970-94) and put them on the map. They found that the mortality rate from this cancer was much lower in the south than in the north. The lowest death rates were in New Mexico, Utah, Arizona and Texas and amounted to approximately 8.89-15.02 deaths per 100,000 inhabitants. There is one important thing in common between these states - they are very solar states. Also in Mississippi, Alabama and Georgia the map looked similar. Essentially, all these states are at a similar latitude. In other words, they are about a similar distance from the equator. And this distance is already short. This is vital because if we are relatively close to the equator and there is plenty of sunshine, we are more likely to have higher levels of vitamin D than someone living in the north. In the north, on the other hand, the death rates were higher, and in particular in the northeast, it was even 23.21-30.39 deaths per 100,000 inhabitants. One may ask why the Northeast was different from the Northwest. It should be remembered that not only vitamin D determines whether someone will have cancer or not. However, it could be influenced by arctic air masses and the cold Labrador current flowing next to this coast. The second reason might be sulfate air pollution caused by burning coal for energy, for which there was a huge demand in this region. This, simply, blocks the UVB rays necessary for the production of vitamin D. In conclusion, in the South, where the possibility of vitamin D production is higher, there was a lower colon cancer mortality than in the North, where the possibility of natural vitamin D production is limited. As I will soon show, this relationship also applied to other types of cancer.

Freedman DM, Looker AC, Chang SC, Graubard BI. **Prospective study of serum vitamin D and cancer mortality in the United States**. J Natl Cancer Inst 2007;99:1594–602.

A total of 16,818 participants in the Third National Health and Nutrition Examination Survey was followed from 1988-1994 through 2000. The researchers concluded that "colorectal cancer mortality was inversely related to serum 25(OH)D level, with levels 80 nmol/L (32ng/ml) or higher associated with a 72% risk reduction compared with lower than 50 nmol/L (20 ng/ml)."

Gorham, Edward Doerr et al. **"Optimal vitamin D status for colorectal cancer prevention: a quantitative meta analysis."** American journal of preventive medicine 32 3 (2007): 210-6 .

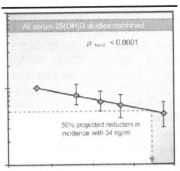

A meta-analysis of five studies found that when our vitamin D levels were 34 ng/ml or higher, we had a 50% lower risk of colorectal cancer than when our vitamin D levels were 12 ng/ml or less.

Yuan, Chen et al. **"Plasma 25-Hydroxyvitamin D Levels and Survival in Patients with Advanced or Metastatic Colorectal Cancer**: Findings from CALGB/SWOG 80405 (Alliance)." Clinical Cancer Research 25 (2019): 7497 - 7505.

In this 2019 study, scientists wanted to examine the relationship between vitamin D levels and overall survival (OS) and progression-free survival (PFS) in patients with advanced or metastatic colorectal cancer. They took blood samples from 1,041 patients. At the start of the study, 63% of patients had vitamin D levels below 20 ng/ml. In addition, 31% of patients had a 25(OH)D3 metabolite level within 20-30 ng/ml. This means that over 94% of patients had vitamin D levels below 30 ng/ml. The researchers noted that higher plasma 25(OH)D levels were associated with improved overall survival and progression-free survival in patients with advanced or metastatic colorectal cancer. They concluded that in these cases the administration of vitamin D is warranted.

Zhang, Lin et al. "**Association between blood circulating vitamin D and colorectal cancer risk in Asian countries**: a systematic review and dose-response meta-analysis." BMJ Open 9 (2019): n. pag.

Zhang, et al, in this publication found that a 16 ng/ml increase in blood vitamin D levels was associated with a 21% lower risk of colorectal cancer. They also mentioned a meta-analysis which showed that risk of colorectal cancer per 10 ng/ml increment in blood circulating vitamin D levels is 26% lower.

Garland, C.F., & Gorham, E.D. (2017). **Dose-response of serum 25-hydroxyvitamin D in association with risk of colorectal cancer**: A meta-analysis. The Journal of Steroid Biochemistry and Molecular Biology, 168, 1-8.

"For example, individuals with a 25(OH)D concentration of 50 ng/ml had an approximately 60% lower risk of colorectal cancer than those with a concentration of 5ng/ml. Those with a 25(OH)D concentration of 30ng/ml had a 33% lower risk than those with a concentration of 5ng/ml. The inverse association between serum 25(OH)D and risk of colorectal cancer overall was strong and statistically significant. There also was a mostly linear dose response relationship between serum 25(OH)D and risk of colorectal cancer when all studies were combined. No study reported significant adverse effects, and there was no evidence of publication bias." - highly regarded researchers Cedric F. Garland and Edward D. Gorham concluded in this meta-analysis that the desired level of vitamin D3 for the prevention of colorectal cancer is over 50 ng/ml. I will mention here that unfortunately most people have vitamin D levels below those 50 ng/ml. In people who already have cancer, this deficiency is even more significant.

Breast cancer

In the case of breast cancer, it is estimated that one in eight women will have this type of cancer. Later in this book I will point out that iodine deficiency in particular plays a big role here. However, as it turns out, vitamin D is no less important. As one study will show, the risk of breast cancer may be reduced by up to 83%. Importantly, vitamin D levels must also be high enough for this to happen. Again, few people have such levels of this vitamin.

The aforementioned scientists Dr. Grant and Dr. Garland found that the situation with the breast cancer mortality rates on the map of the US looked similar to the one for colon cancer. Here, too, in the south, the death rate was lower compared to the north. The role of vitamin D cannot be ruled out in this case as well, because such a significant correlation has been found also by other scientists.

Mohr, Sharif Burgette et al. **"Relationship between Low Ultraviolet B Irradiance and Higher Breast Cancer Risk in 107 Countries."** The Breast Journal 14 (2008): n. pag.

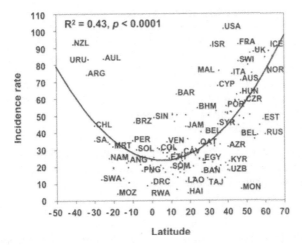

This graph shows the latitude and incidence of breast cancer. As it turns out, the farther from the equator, the higher the incidence. For example, New Zealand (NZL), far in the southern hemisphere of the world, has a high incidence of breast cancer. The same is true for Iceland (ICE), which is far from the equator in the Northern Hemisphere. On the other hand, there are countries such as Mozambique, Rwanda and Haiti that have low rates of breast cancer. All of these countries are close to the equator.

Lowe, Lorraine C. et al. **"Plasma 25-hydroxy vitamin D concentrations, vitamin D receptor genotype and breast cancer risk in a UK Caucasian population."** European journal of cancer 41 8 (2005): 1164-9 .

Scientists have studied the relationship between 25(OH)D3 levels and the incidence of breast cancer in the United Kingdom population. They concluded that when the vitamin D level is 48 ng/ml, the risk of breast cancer is 50% lower compared to the lowest quartile. However, if this level is 60 ng/ml, the risk will be reduced by 83%.

Goodwin, Pamela J. et al. **"Prognostic effects of 25-hydroxyvitamin D levels in early breast cancer."** Journal of clinical oncology : official journal of the American Society of Clinical Oncology 27 23 (2009): 3757-63 .

512 women with early stages of breast cancer were included in this study. Mean follow-up was 11.6 years. If vitamin D levels were above 28.8 ng/ml, the risk of death was more than 40% lower than in women who had levels below 20 ng/ml. It is also worth mentioning that in this study, as many as 76% of the study participants had vitamin D levels below 30 ng/ml. This result would therefore be similar to that obtained in previous studies and indicate that insufficient levels of this vitamin are very common in people with cancer.

Madden, J M et al. **"De novo vitamin D supplement use post-diagnosis is associated with breast cancer survival."** Breast Cancer Research and Treatment 172 (2018): 179-190.

In this study of 5,417 women with a record of invasive breast cancer aged 50-80 years, 2,581 women were administered vitamin D. There was a 20% reduction in breast cancer-specific mortality in vitamin D patients (modeled as a time-varying variable) compared to the group that did not take vitamin D. However, if vitamin D was initiated soon after the breast cancer diagnosis (within 6 months) there was a 49% reduction in mortality.

Ovarian Cancer

Ovarian cancer is the fifth leading cause of cancer death. The most common is epithelial ovarian cancer which represents 90% of all cases. It is often diagnosed at an advanced stage in most patients with a survival rate of less than 40% at 5 years. Hence, it is worth taking a closer look at this cancer and whether it is not associated with vitamin D deficiency. We'll start again with correlation and move on to other studies.

The ovarian cancer mortality map created by dr. Grand and dr. Garland looked similar to the ones shown earlier. In almost all southern states, the death rate due to ovarian cancer was 4.85-6.58 compared to the northern states where the death rate was even 9.32-11.16 per 100,000 inhabitants. In other words, the death rate was mainly higher at higher latitudes, where the ability to achieve adequate vitamin D levels through sun exposure is significantly reduced.

Lefkowitz, Eva S and Cedric F. Garland. "**Sunlight, vitamin D, and ovarian cancer mortality rates in US women.**" International journal of epidemiology 23 6 (1994): 1133-6 .

In the above similar publication, scientists investigated the fact that ovarian cancer mortality in counties containing the 100 largest US cities is higher in northern than southern latitudes. In their analysis, they also took into account the presence of ozone and sulfur dioxide in the atmosphere in certain regions as it absorbs radiation. The study clearly indicated that sunlight may be a protective factor for ovarian cancer mortality.

Walentowicz-Sadłecka, Małgorzata et al. "**25(OH)D3 in patients with ovarian cancer and its correlation with survival.**" Clinical biochemistry 45 18 (2012): 1568-72 .

One study aimed to examine, inter alia, the association between 25(OH)D concentration in ovarian cancer patients and overall 5-year survival. 72 epithelial ovarian cancer patients aged 37-79 were enrolled in the study group. The level of vitamin D was measured in this group as well as in the group of 65 healthy women aged 35-65 years. In cancer patients the level of vitamin D was 12.5 ± 7.75 ng/ml, whereas in the reference group it was 22.4 ± 6.5 ng/ml. The studied group of sick patients was then divided into two groups. As it turned out, the overall 5-year survival rate was significantly higher in the group of patients with vitamin D levels higher than 10 ng/ml than in the group with patients with levels lower than 10 ng/ml.

Kitami, Kazuhisa et al. **"Peritoneal Restoration by Repurposing Vitamin D Inhibits Ovarian Cancer Dissemination via Blockade of the TGF-β1/Thrombospondin-1 Axis."** Matrix biology : journal of the International Society for Matrix Biology (2022): n. pag.

"Vitamin D restores cancer-associated mesothelial cells to an epithelial state with normalization of THBS1 expression in preclinical models that mimic cancerous peritonitis in vivo."
This tumor often metastasizes to the peritoneum. The mesothelial cells lining it are supposed to interfere with this. This May 2022 publication pointed to an important mechanism by which vitamin D may prevent metastasis. To explain this briefly, cancer cells produce the TGF-ß1 protein. This protein causes an increase in the production of another protein, thrombospondin-1 (THBS1). We usually find elevated amounts of this protein in the later stages of ovarian cancer. Thrombospondin-1 allows cancer cells to adhere to the peritoneum and form a metastasis. Vitamin D, on the other hand, inhibits the production of thrombospondin caused by more TGF-ß1 protein. In this way, vitamin D can prevent metastasis and prove essential in treatment.

Prostate cancer

Of course, colorectal, breast and ovarian cancer are not the only cancers in which vitamin D shows anti-cancer properties. Also in the case of prostate cancer, studies have shown that higher blood vitamin D levels are associated with a reduced risk of death due to this disease. Supplementation with this vitamin, in turn, correlates with lower prostate-specific antigen (PSA) levels, which, when elevated, may indicate the presence of prostate cancer. Moreover, studies have found that people with prostate cancer, like those with other cancers, have low levels of vitamin D. But that's not all.

Bao BY, Yao J, Lee YF. **1alpha, 25-dihydroxyvitamin D3 suppresses interleukin-8-mediated prostate cancer cell angiogenesis**. Carcinogenesis. 2006;27(9):1883–93.

This publication indicated that vitamin D can prevent prostate cancer progression by interrupting interleukin-8 signaling

(IL-8). IL-8 may play a role in tumor progression and affect the increase in angiogenesis (growth of blood vessels from the existing vasculature, in this case a cancer). Hence, vitamin D may have the effect of reducing or inhibiting the progression of prostate cancer.

Grant, W.B. (2002). **An estimate of premature cancer mortality in the U.S. due to inadequate doses of solar ultraviolet-B radiation**. Cancer, 94.

Results from another study: "The findings of the current study confirm previous results that solar UV-B radiation is associated with reduced risk of cancer of the breast, colon, ovary, and prostate as well as non-Hodgkin lymphoma. Eight additional malignancies were found to exhibit an inverse correlation between mortality rates and UV-B radiation: bladder, esophageal, kidney, lung, pancreatic, rectal, stomach, and corpus uteri."

Thyroid cancer

Thyroid cancer affects almost three times more women than men. Unlike other cancers, it is also a cancer that is diagnosed more often in younger people. Although it is rarely associated with vitamin D by the common people, such a relationship has already been found by many scientific publications.

Zhao, Jun-yu et al. **"Vitamin D deficiency as a risk factor for thyroid cancer: A meta-analysis of case-control studies."** Nutrition 57 (2019): 5-11.

For this reason, the authors of the above publication decided to conduct a meta-analysis examining the relationship between vitamin D levels and the risk of thyroid cancer. To this end, they analyzed 14 available scientific publications on this topic. They found that people who are deficient in vitamin D have an increased risk of thyroid cancer by 30% and generally lower serum 25(OH)D levels are associated with increased risk for thyroid cancer.

Lung cancer

Lung cancer is the second most common cancer worldwide. It is the most common cancer in men and the second most common cancer in women. In 2020 alone, 2.2 million new cases of lung cancer were detected. Therefore, it is critical to stop this tragedy. Studies have shown that here, too, vitamin D may prove to be helpful in the prevention and fight against cancer. Here are some of them:

Chen, Wanqing et al. "**Relationship between cancer mortality/ incidence and ambient ultraviolet B irradiance in China**." Cancer Causes & Control 21 (2010): 1701-1709.

Researchers investigated the relationship between incidence and mortality from a number of cancers and ultraviolet irradiance in China. Mortality rates for cancers such as esophagus, stomach, colon and rectum, liver, lung, breast, and bladder were inversely correlated with solar UVB. Interestingly, in the case of lung cancer, there was the strongest inverse correlation with an estimated 12% fall per 10 mW/(nm m(2)) increase in UVB. The authors concluded: "Mortality from all cancers together and most major cancers in China was inversely associated with solar UVB. These associations were similar to those observed in a number of populations of European origin."

Zhang L, Wang S, Che X, Li X: **Vitamin D and Lung Cancer Risk: A Comprehensive Review and Meta-Analysis**. Cell Physiol Biochem 2015;36:299-305. doi: 10.1159/000374072

The above meta-analysis examining the relationship between lung cancer and vitamin D was based on 12 studies and included 288,778 participants. It indicates that high vitamin D status is associated with decreased risk of lung cancer. Vitamin D may induce apoptosis (process of programmed cell death) in small cell lung carcinoma cell lines. Moreover, due to this vitamin, there may also be an additive decrease in cell proliferation (growth of cells). Vitamin D has the ability to prevent angiogenesis (process of new blood vessel formation). In addition, we have also learned based on animal models that vitamin D can inhibit the metastatic growth of lung cancer cells.

Skin cancer

For a long time it was believed that skin cancer was caused by exposure to the sun. Many doctors and people still believe it. However, it seems quite the opposite. Not only is skin cancer not caused by the sun, but a lack of sun can contribute to its formation. In this, vitamin D deficiency may play a major role. We know some of the mechanisms by which vitamin D can act as a protective agent, and we have studies showing that low vitamin D levels are associated with increased mortality from skin cancer.

Muralidhar, Sathya et al. **"Vitamin D-VDR signaling inhibits Wnt/beta-catenin-mediated melanoma progression and promotes anti-tumor immunity."** Cancer research (2019): n. pag.

"Vitamin D-VDR (VDR - vitamin D receptor) signaling contributes to controlling pro-proliferative/immunosuppressive Wnt/β-catenin signaling in melanoma and this is associated with less metastatic disease and stronger host immune responses. This is evidence of a causal relationship between vitamin D-VDR signaling and melanoma survival, which should be explored as a therapeutic target in primary resistance to checkpoint blockade. (...) VDR expression could potentially be used as a biomarker to stratify patients with melanoma that may respond better to immunotherapy."

When the Wnt/β-catenin pathway is active, the immune response is suppressed to counteract tumor formation. This pathway also promotes cell proliferation and tumor growth. Suppression of this pathway by vitamin D reduces the rate of tumor growth and metastasis and also supports host immunity.

Timerman D, McEnery-Stonelake M, Joyce CJ, et al. **Vitamin D deficiency is associated with a worse prognosis in metastatic melanoma**. Oncotarget. 2017;8(4):6873-6882. doi:10.18632/oncotarget.14316

The authors of this publication investigated the relationship between vitamin D levels and prognosis in metastatic melanoma. 252 people with histopathology-confirmed melanoma and measured 25(OH)D levels within one year after diagnosis were included in the study. In patients with stage IV metastatic melanoma, a vitamin D level below 20 ng/ml was associated with significantly worse melanoma-specific mortality. It was similar in patients who initially had a deficiency of this vitamin, and then the level decreased or increased, but was still below 20 ng/ml. These patients had also significantly worse outcomes compared to patients with 25(OH)D levels above 20 ng/ml.

Berwick, Marianne et al. **"Sun exposure and mortality from melanoma."** Journal of the National Cancer Institute 97 3 (2005): 195-9.

Associated with increased death	Associated with decreased death
Melanoma Thickness	Sunburn
Mitoses	High intermittent sun exposure
Ulceration	Skin awareness histories
Anatomic location on the head and neck	Solar elastosis

The results of the analysis of risk factors for dying from melanoma clearly showed that "Sunburn, high intermittent sun exposure, skin awareness histories, and solar elastosis (condition due to prolonged sun exposure) were statistically significantly inversely associated with death from melanoma. Melanoma thickness, mitoses (cell division), ulceration, and anatomic location on the head and neck were statistically significantly positively associated with melanoma death." Hence, as it turns out, and as can be seen, all sun exposure is associated with a reduced mortality from skin cancer. This is evidence of the protective effect of the sun. However, of course, staying in the sun until it comes to sunburn is not recommended. It will be optimal for no more than half an hour in full sun. But more on that a little later.

Lindqvist, Pelle G. et al. **"Avoidance of sun exposure as a risk factor for major causes of death: a competing risk analysis of the Melanoma in Southern Sweden cohort."** Journal of Internal Medicine 280 (2016): 375 - 387.

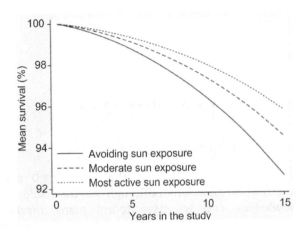

The above very large study involving nearly 30,000 selected at random women aged 35-64 years investigated the correlation between sun exposure and all-cause mortality. These women were followed prospectively for 20 years with 2,545 deaths recorded during this time. Finally, this study showed (as seen in the graph) that people who had active sun exposure habits also had a longer life expectancy than people who avoided sun exposure. More precisely, people with the highest sun exposure could have a life expectancy of up to 2 years longer than sun-avoiding people. This study, thus, goes beyond skin cancer or other cancers, embraces overall and shows that those who spend the most time in the sun also live the longest.

CHAPTER 2:
INFECTIONS

We have known for some time that vitamin D plays an important role in infections (although we have seldom used this knowledge), and we have found many mechanisms of vitamin D's action then. Vitamin D has a modulating function in both the adaptive and innate immune system. Vitamin D induces production of antimicrobial peptides by macrophages, monocytes, keratinocytes, epithelial, intestinal, lung, and corneal cells. In the case of the first two (macrophages and monocytes), this contributes to the intensification of chemotaxis (directed migration of cells) and autophagy (which has many key functions). In epithelial, intestinal, lung, and corneal cells this enhances physical barrier function. Moreover, vitamin D can inhibit the production of pro-inflammatory cytokines such as IL-12, IFN-γ, IL-6, IL-8, TNF-α, and IL-9. And, on the other hand, enhance the production of anti-inflammatory cytokines such as IL-4, IL-5, and IL-10. These are, of course, not all of the vitamin D's mechanisms of action, nor are most of them. But to summarize it briefly, vitamin D modulates antiviral and antibacterial inflammatory immune responses. This is so important because various types of infections accompany our lives all the time. In a moment, we'll look at these different infections and see how they relate to vitamin D. Let me mention now that this relationship will turn out to be strong. We will start with the still popular COVID-19, a correlation study and then other studies.

COVID-19

Walrand, S. (2021). **Autumn COVID-19 surge dates in Europe correlated to latitudes, not to temperature-humidity, pointing**

to vitamin D as contributing factor. Scientific Reports, 11.

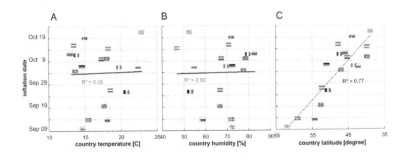

In this publication, authors investigated the correlations between COVID-19 surge dates in Europe and latitude, temperature and humidity. There was no correlation whatsoever in the case of humidity (middle graph). Similarly, as you can see in the left graph above, there was no correlation between COVID-19 surge dates and temperature. However, in the case of latitude, this correlation was almost perfect (right graph). COVID-19 surges began the earliest in Finland or Sweden (i.s. in the north) and were the latest in Greece or Spain (in the south of the continent). Solar radiation was important therefore here, and if so, vitamin D could also play a large role. However, it cannot be ignored that not only vitamin D is associated with solar radiation. Part of the spectrum of solar radiation is UV radiation. As we know, UVB contributes to the production of vitamin D, which is wonderful for our health and excellent in the case of infections (more on that in a moment). Visible light, in turn, affects Circadian Rhythm. The infrared light (also a part of solar radiation) influences melatonin, which is a powerful antioxidant. Therefore, it is important to remember that solar radiation is not only about vitamin D. Apart from taking care of the proper level of this vitamin, it is worth going out in the sun (also during disease). Now let's move on to studies exploring the link between COVID-19 and vitamin D.

Jain, Anshul Kumar et al. "**Analysis of vitamin D level among asymptomatic and critically ill COVID-19 patients and its correlation with inflammatory markers.**" Scientific Reports 10

(2020): n. pag.

In this publication, scientists wanted to analyze the level of 25(OH)D in COVID-19 patients and its impact on the disease severity. Participants were COVID-19 patients of age group 30–60 years. Out of 154 participants, 91 were asymptomatic (first group) and 63 were severely ill (second group). The mean level of vitamin D was 27.89 ng/ml in the first group and 14.35 ng/ml in second, the difference was highly significant. The prevalence of vitamin D deficiency was 32.96% and 96.82% respectively in the first group and the second group. In addition, levels of various inflammatory markers (IL-6, ferritin, TNFα) were higher in patients deficient in vitamin D. The same applies to the fatality rate which was high in vitamin D deficient (21% vs 3.1%).

Dror, Amiel A. et al. "**Pre-infection 25-hydroxyvitamin D3 levels and association with severity of COVID-19 illness.**" PLoS ONE 17 (2021): n. pag.

This study aimed to examine the correlations between vitamin D and both risk of infection with SARS-CoV-2 and poorer clinical outcomes. Importantly, vitamin D levels in patients were checked 14 to 730 days prior to COVID-19 diagnosis. In this way, we can rule out the claim that the disease itself contributed to the vitamin D deficiency and not the other way around, i.e. the deficiency of this vitamin contributed to the infection. Thus, 253 individuals with pre-infection 25(OH)D levels were included in the study. 133 people had vitamin D levels below 20 ng/ml. 36 people had 25(OH)D levels between 20 and 30 ng/ml. 44 subjects had levels between 30 and 40 ng/ml. And 40 people had the level above 40 ng/ml. As it turned out, 87.4% of patients with severe or critical disease had vitamin D levels below 20 ng/ml. On the other hand, vitamin D levels below 20 ng/ml were reported in only 34.3% of people with mild or moderate disease. Consequently, the calculations showed that patients with 25(OH)D levels below 20 ng/ml are 14 times more likely to have severe or critical disease. Additionally, the mortality rate for patients with vitamin D deficiency was 25.6%. In contrast, in patients with sufficient vitamin D levels, the mortality rate was 2.3% (p < 0.001).

Borsche, Lorenz et al. "COVID-19 **Mortality Risk Correlates**

Inversely with Vitamin D3 Status, and a Mortality Rate Close to Zero Could Theoretically Be Achieved at 50 ng/mL 25(OH)D3: Results of a Systematic Review and Meta-Analysis." Nutrients 13 (2021): n. pag.

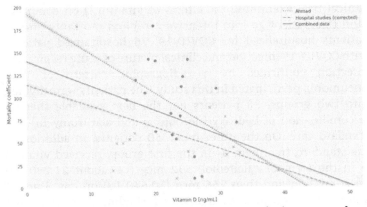

In this systematic review and meta-analysis, researchers investigated the relationship between vitamin D and COVID-19 mortality. Patients' 25(OH)D levels were reported either pre-infection or on the day of hospital admission. This suggests that vitamin D was not lowered by infection. The median vitamin D levels were 23.2 ng/ml. There was a strong negative correlation between vitamin D levels and mortality from this disease. As regression suggested a theoretical point of zero mortality at approximately 50 ng/ml. This can be seen well in the graph above. The undotted line is the combination of hospital and population data. As you can see, the mortality disappeared at levels above 50 ng/ml. The researchers concluded the results of the study as follows: "The datasets provide strong evidence that low D3 is a predictor rather than just a side effect of the infection. Despite ongoing vaccinations, we recommend raising serum 25(OH)D levels to above 50 ng/ml to prevent or mitigate new outbreaks due to escape mutations or decreasing antibody activity."

Entrenas Castillo, Marta et al. ""**Effect of calcifediol treatment and best available therapy versus best available therapy on intensive care unit admission and mortality among patients**

hospitalized for COVID-19: A pilot randomized clinical study"." The Journal of Steroid Biochemistry and Molecular Biology 203 (2020): 105751 - 105751.

It was the parallel pilot randomized open label, a double-masked clinical trial examining the effects of vitamin D on condition (will this patient go into intensive care) and mortality among patients hospitalized for COVID-19. 76 hospitalized patients with COVID-19 infection and clinical picture of acute respiratory infection confirmed by a radiographic pattern of viral pneumonia participated in this study. The patients were divided into two groups. 26 patients got the best available therapy (a combination of hydroxychloroquine and azithromycin) and standard care. On the other hand, 50 patients, in addition to the standard treatment as in the first group, received vitamin D in the form of calcifediol; 532 mcg (i.e. about 21,280 IU) on admission and then 266 mcg (10,640 IU) on day 3 and 7 and then weekly until discharge or ICU admission. Calcifediol was used because it raises vitamin D levels very quickly, unlike cholecalciferol (found e.g. in supplements) which needs at least a few days to be metabolized into its active form. As for the effects, 2% of 50 patients treated with calcifediol required admission to the intensive care unit. On the other hand, of the 26 patients not treated with calcifediol, as many as 50% required admission to the ICU. Moreover, of the patients treated with calcifediol, no one died and everyone left the clinic without complications. In patients untreated with calcifediol and admitted to the ICU, two people died. Although it was a fairly small study, it was conducted very well and the results were significant.

Lakkireddy, M., Gadiga, S.G., Malathi, R.D. et al. **Impact of daily high dose oral vitamin D therapy on the inflammatory markers in patients with COVID 19 disease.** Sci Rep 11, 10641 (2021). https://doi.org/10.1038/s41598-021-90189-4

In this study, researchers wanted to investigate the effect of vitamin D on various inflammatory markers of COVID-19 (N/L ratio, CRP, LDH, IL6, Ferritin). Patients had vitamin D deficiency with the mean of 16 ng/ml. The division was made into two groups. One group was getting 60,000 IU/day of vitamin D for 8 to 10 days (depending upon their BMI) plus standard treatment. The other group only got standard treatment. 44 people from the first group and 43 people from the second group completed the study. As it turned out, there was a highly significant reduction of all the measured inflammatory markers in the vitamin D group. What is crucial, the level of 25(OH)D in this group increased to 89 ng/ml. On the other hand, in the group without vitamin D, the reduction of inflammatory markers was insignificant. Authors stated that therapeutic improvement occurred in the range of 80-100 ng/ml and without any side effects. Furthermore, they suggested that this therapy could be added to the existing treatment protocols of COVID-19.

Although, having lived for the past over two years, one might believe that we are only at risk of COVID-19, this is not the case. Other infections are still present, people get sick and sometimes die. It is important to be aware of this. Therefore, now we will review studies that also look at other infections and our vitamin.

Other common infections

Sabetta, James R. et al. "**Serum 25-Hydroxyvitamin D and the Incidence of Acute Viral Respiratory Tract Infections in Healthy Adults.**" PLoS ONE 5 (2010): n. pag.

In this prospective cohort study, researchers wanted to investigate the relationship between 25(OH)D levels and the incidence of acute viral respiratory tract infections (ARTIs). To this end, they measured vitamin D levels over the fall and winter of 198 healthy adults. As it turned out, only 17% of people who maintained 25(OH)D levels above 38 ng/ml throughout the study developed ARTIs. On the other hand, when the vitamin D level was below 38 ng/ml, the incidence of ARTIs was 45%. Thus, levels above 38 ng/ml were significantly associated with twofold reduction in risk of developing ARTIs. Moreover, a higher level was associated with a marked reduction in the percentages of days ill.

Other studies, in turn, found that the incidence rate of respiratory tract infections decreased by 7% with an increase in 25(OH)D levels by 10 nmol/l (4ng/ml).

Martineau, Adrian R. et al. "**Vitamin D supplementation to**

prevent acute respiratory tract infections: systematic review and meta-analysis of individual participant data." The BMJ 356 (2017): n. pag.

In this meta-analysis, including 25 eligible randomized controlled trials and over 10,933 participants, the authors assessed the overall effect of vitamin D supplementation on risk of acute respiratory tract infections. Among all participants vitamin D supplementation (in every form, including bolus doses e.g. once a month) reduced the risk of acute respiratory tract infection by 12%. However, as has been shown, better effects were found as a result of daily or weekly vitamin D supplementation without bolus doses. In this case, the protection effect increased to 19%. What's more, in subjects who at baseline had vitamin D levels below 25 nmol/L (10 ng/ml), when this level was corrected with supplementation, the risk of acute respiratory tract infections was reduced by 70%.

Bergman, Peter et al. "**Vitamin D supplementation to patients with frequent respiratory tract infections: a post hoc analysis of a randomized and placebo-controlled trial.**" BMC Research Notes 8 (2015): n. pag.

The aim of this post hoc analysis of a randomized and placebo-controlled trial was to test whether vitamin D reduces the number of respiratory tract infections (RTIs). 124 adult patients with a high burden of RTIs participated in the study. They got 4,000 IU of vitamin D for a year. In the primary study, it was found that the total numbers of respiratory bacterial cultures were reduced by approximately 50% in the vitamin D group. Additionally, in the same group, the antibiotic consumption was reduced by 60%. In a post-hoc analysis, in turn, it was found that vitamin D significantly increased the probability of staying infection free during the study period. The total number of RTIs was also reduced in this group. Additionally, the time to the first RTI was significantly extended.

Han, Jenny E et al. "**High dose vitamin D administration in ventilated intensive care unit patients: A pilot double blind randomized controlled trial.**" Journal of Clinical & Translational Endocrinology 4 (2016): 59 - 65.

In this pilot, double blind randomized control trial researchers examined the effects of vitamin D on mechanically ventilated adult intensive care unit patients. The subjects were given a placebo, 50,000 IU of vitamin D or 100,000 IU vitamin D daily for the next 5 days. So it was 250,000IU and 500,000IU respectively. After seven days, the mean serum 25(OH)D level in the 250,000 IU supplementation group rose to 45 ng/ml. In the group that received a total of 500,000 IU of vitamin D, it was 55 ng/ml. In the placebo group the initial 21 ng/ml remained. As it turned out, there was a significant decrease in hospital length of stay in the groups supplementing vitamin D. It was 36 days in the control group, 25 days in the 250,000 IU supplementation group and 18 days in the 500,000 IU supplementation group (i.e. two times less than in the control group).

Zhou, Yun et al. "**The association between vitamin D deficiency and community-acquired pneumonia.**" Medicine 98 (2019): n. pag.

The above meta-analysis, including eight observational studies involving 20,966 subjects, evaluated the relationship between vitamin D deficiency and pneumonia. People deficient in vitamin D (25(OH)D levels < 20 ng/ml) in this meta-analysis experienced a significantly increased risk of community-acquired pneumonia (CAP) of up to 64%. In addition, there was found a decrease in vitamin D levels of – 5.63 ng/ml in people with CAP compared to healthy individuals.

Urashima, Mitsuyoshi et al. "**Randomized trial of vitamin D supplementation to prevent seasonal influenza A in schoolchildren.**" The American journal of clinical nutrition 91 5 (2010): 1255-60.

In this randomized, double-blind, placebo-controlled trial, the authors wanted to evaluate the effect of vitamin D on the incidence of seasonal influenza A in schoolchildren. 334 children were divided into two groups of 167 people each. One group got 1,200 IU of vitamin D while the other group got a placebo. In the vitamin D group, 18 out of 167 (10.8%) children got influenza A. In the placebo group, however, it was 31 out of 167 (18.6%). This means that vitamin D reduced the relative risk of getting influenza A by 42%. Moreover, vitamin D in children with a previous diagnosis of asthma reduced the relative risk of asthma attacks by over 83% (2 vs 12 cases).

Zhou, Jian et al. **"Preventive Effects of Vitamin D on Seasonal Influenza A in Infants:** A Multicenter, Randomized, Open, Controlled Clinical Trial." The Pediatric Infectious Disease Journal 37 (2018): 749–754.

This study was designed to evaluate the effects of vitamin D on preventing influenza A in 400 infants 3–12 months old. Half of the infants received the lower dose of 400 IU vitamin D daily for 4 months and the other half the higher dose of 1,200 IU daily for 4 months. There were 121 cases of influenza A infection, 65% of which were in the group with the lower dose of vitamin D and 35% in the higher dose group. So already in this aspect there was a significant difference between the groups. What's more, the median duration of a fever in the higher-dose vitamin D group was significantly shorter than that in the lower-dose vitamin D group. Exactly the same was the case with coughing. There was a significant difference between the duration of the cough with less of it in the 1200 IU group. Also, the median duration of wheezing was lower in the group receiving the higher dose of vitamin D compared to the group receiving the lower dose. The scientists concluded that "high-dose vitamin D (1200 IU) is suitable for the prevention of seasonal influenza as evidenced by rapid relief from symptoms, rapid decrease in viral loads and disease recovery. In addition, high-dose vitamin D is probably safe for infants." This study therefore offered a solution to the worries and anxiety of many mothers and fathers about their children's illness. This solution is vitamin D, which can prevent their children from catching influenza A, among others. If only more of them were aware of this...

Deng, Qifei et al. **"Vitamin D and Urinary Tract Infection: A Systematic Review and Meta-Analysis".** Annals of clinical and laboratory science 49 1 (2019): 134-142.

For this systematic review and meta-analysis from 2019, 9 studies were included with 1921 participants, of which 580 were diagnosed with urinary tract infections (UTI). The analysis showed that vitamin D insufficiency was associated with a significantly increased risk of having a UTI. The mean 25(OH)D level was also significantly lower in the UTI group than in the control group. The mean difference between the groups was as high as 9.60 ng/ml. Moreover, this level differed by 10.40 ng/ml when the UTI cases were compared with the control group in children.

Tekin, Mehmet et al. **"The Association between Vitamin D Levels and Urinary Tract Infection in Children."** Hormone Research in Paediatrics 83 (2015): 198 - 203.

In this study, the authors wanted to investigate the relationship between vitamin D and urinary tract infection (UTI) among children. To this end, they measured the level of 25(OH)D in 82 children experiencing a first episode of UTI and 64 healthy control children. The mean serum levels of 25(OH)D among children with UTI were 11.7 ng/ml and were significantly lower than in the control group. There, the mean vitamin D level was 27.6 ng/ml. Interestingly, in patients with acute pyelonephritis (pyelonephritis is often a complication of an ascending urinary tract infection), the mean level of vitamin D was even lower and amounted to 8.6 ng/ml. The authors concluded that 25(OH)D levels below 20 ng/ml were associated with UTI in children.

Çayır, Atilla et al. **"Serum vitamin D levels in children with recurrent otitis media."** European Archives of Oto-Rhino-Laryngology 271 (2013): 689-693.

In this study, researchers examined vitamin D levels in children with recurrent otitis media, compared them with levels in healthy children, and also checked the effect of vitamin D therapy on the risk of recurrence of this disease. Eighty-four children (1-5 years of age) diagnosed with recurrent otitis media and one hundred-and-eight healthy children were included. The mean level of vitamin D in the study group was 11.4 ng/ml and the level below 20 ng/ml affected almost 70% of children. In the group of healthy children, however, the mean level of vitamin D was 29.2 ng/ml and the level below 20 ng/ml concerned 30% of children. Additionally, vitamin D supplementation in deficient children with recurrent otitis media was shown to be beneficial.

Schwalfenberg GK. **Treatment of Infectious Mononucleosis**

with High Dose Vitamin D3 in Three Cases. Ann Nutr Disord & Ther. 2021; 8(1): 1068.

This publication described single clinical practice of documented infectious mononucleosis treated with high dose vitamin D. Three people were quite ill with worsening symptoms daily prior to getting vitamin D. I will briefly present these cases.

Case 1. A 17-year-old woman had symptoms such as fever, headache, sore throat, lymphadenopathy, periorbital edema and extreme fatigue, among others. Despite taking 2,000 IU throughout the winter, this did not seem to have a significant impact. She saw a pediatrician with suspected angina and got medication. However, the symptoms continued to worsen. Vitamin D therapy was initiated. The patient received 50,000 IU of vitamin D daily for three days and then 10,000 IU daily for one month. After five days there was a significant improvement in fatigue and concentration. Furthermore, within 10 days she returned to her normal premorbid. After a month, her vitamin D levels increased to 81 ng/ml.

Case 2. Another case was a 17-year-old man with fever, headache, sore throat with significant lymphadenopathy, splenomegaly and significant difficulty swallowing. Due to the worsening of symptoms and difficulty swallowing, treatment with vitamin D was initiated. The male was given 50,000 IU daily for 4 days followed by 10,000 IU for a month. After six days, there was a significant improvement in energy and he was able to return to school. The fatigue ceased within two weeks. His 25(OH)D level after 4 weeks was 35 ng/ml.

Leaving aside for a while. In this example, we can see that relatively high doses do not always lead to rapid increases in vitamin D levels. Sometimes, in some people and in various disease entities, much more vitamin D is needed to reach desired levels.

Case 3. The last case is a 16-year-old man with very similar symptoms as before. Before his illness, his 25(OH)D level was 17 ng/ml. The patient received 50,000 IU for 4 days and then 10,000 IU daily for a month. His symptoms resolved within a few days which allowed him to return to school without having fatigue. The lymphadenopathy also resolved within two weeks.

The patient continued supplementation with vitamin D in a dose of 8,000-10,000 IU for the next three months, which contributed to an increase in the level of vitamin D to 135 ng/ml.

CHAPTER 3:
INFLAMMATION

Inflammation is what accompanies almost all diseases. I already mentioned in the previous chapter that vitamin D is able to inhibit the production of pro-inflammatory cytokines (IL-12, IFN-γ, IL-6, IL-8, TNF-α, IL-9) and enhance the production of anti-inflammatory cytokines (IL-4, IL-5, IL-10). However, vitamin D can do even more.

Tabatabaeizadeh, Seyed-Amir et al. **"High Dose Supplementation of Vitamin D Affects Measures of Systemic Inflammation: Reductions in High Sensitivity C-Reactive Protein Level and Neutrophil to Lymphocyte Ratio (NLR) Distribution."** Journal of Cellular Biochemistry 118 (2017): n. pag.

First, let me explain two things. C-reactive protein (CRP) is a protein produced by the liver in response to inflammation. A CRP result within the normal range means that no infection is developing in the patient's body. On the other hand, an elevated CRP result indicates the infection (and therefore also inflammation). Moreover, much higher levels may indicate cancer or rheumatoid diseases, for example. Neutrophil to lymphocyte ratio (NLR) is a widely used reliable and easily available marker of immune response to various infectious and non-infectious stimuli. Its elevated levels may indicate pathological states such as cancer, atherosclerosis, infection, inflammation, stress and psychiatric disorders. If this is already clear, let's move on to what the above study showed. A total of 580 adolescent girls were included and the indicators of systemic inflammation measured, before and after supplementation at a dose of 50,000 IU/week (i.e. about 7142 IU/day) for 9 weeks. At the end, the researchers observed that there was a significant reduction in neutrophil count and CRP level after vitamin

D supplementation, which proved that this vitamin affects measures of systemic inflammation and reduces it.

CHAPTER 4:
AUTOIMMUNE
DISEASE

An autoimmune disease is when the immune system produces antibodies that attack the body's own cells, tissues and organs. Autoimmune diseases can occur almost anywhere in the body. It is estimated that in the United States up to 8% of the population suffers from some kind of autoimmune disease, and this trend is growing worldwide. As you will see shortly, vitamin D is a powerful agent in both the prevention and treatment of these types of diseases. First we will look at it in general and later in the book we will move on to individual diseases of an autoimmune nature.

Hahn, Jill et al. "**Vitamin D and marine omega 3 fatty acid supplementation and incident autoimmune disease: VITAL randomized controlled trial.**" The BMJ 376 (2022): n. pag.

In this large and qualitative randomized controlled trial from 2022, the authors wanted to evaluate the impact of Vitamin D and marine omega 3 fatty acid supplementation on incidence of autoimmune disease. For this purpose 25 871 participants were enrolled and followed for a median of 5.3 years. The division into four groups was made. One group received vitamin D (2000 IU/day) and omega 3 (1g/day), the second group received vitamin D and placebo, the third group received omega 3 and placebo, and the fourth group only received a placebo. The primary endpoint was total confirmed autoimmune disease incidence (such as, but not limited to: rheumatoid arthritis, polymyalgia rheumatica, autoimmune thyroid disease, psoriasis, and inflammatory bowel disease). The levels of 25(OH)D in those taking vitamin D supplementation increased from an average of 29.8 ng/ml to 41.8 ng/ml. When it comes to people taking omega-3 supplements, blood levels increased by 55%.

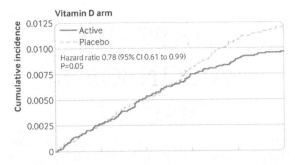

All incident confirmed autoimmune diseases

As we can see in the chart above, in the group supplementing vitamin D over a 5 years period of time the incidence of autoimmune diseases was reduced by 22%. In the case of supplementation with only omega-3, the incidence of autoimmune diseases was reduced by 15% (however not statistically significant). In the group that took both vitamin D and omega-3, this reduction was over 31%. Moreover, when only the last three years of the study were taken into account, the vitamin D group had 39% fewer participants with confirmed autoimmune disease than the placebo group. What is also worth noting, the effect of vitamin D on the reduction of autoimmune diseases also depended on the BMI (Body Mass Index) of the person. The higher this index was, the lower the improvement was. Later I will demonstrate that obese people simply need more vitamin D to achieve the same 25(OH)D level as non obese people.

CHAPTER 5: PARKINSON'S DISEASE

Parkinson's disease is also increasingly considered an autoimmune disease. Its symptoms include, for example, tremor, rigid muscles, slowed movement, speech changes, impaired balance and problems with writing. Vitamin D, as it turns out, can protect against this disease as well. Vitamin D enhances the synthesis of dopamine. And what's more, studies suggest vitamin D has a neuroprotective effect on dopaminergic pathways in the central nervous system. These are some of the possible reasons why the following studies have obtained such results.

Lv, Zheng et al. **"Vitamin D status and Parkinson's disease: a systematic review and meta-analysis."** Neurological Sciences 35 (2014): 1723-1730.

The above scientific publication took into account 1.008 patients and 4.536 controls. They found that people with Parkinson's disease had lower 25(OH)D levels than healthy people. Patients with vitamin D <75 nmol/l (30 ng/ml) had an increased risk of Parkinson's disease. However, patients with vitamin D levels <50 nmol/L (20 ng/ml) have a twofold increased risk of this disease.

Hiller, Amie L et al. **"A randomized, controlled pilot study of the effects of vitamin D supplementation on balance in Parkinson's disease: Does age matter?"** PLoS ONE 13 (2018): n. pag.

In this study, 51 people received 10,000 IU per day or a placebo for 16 weeks. The level of 25(OH)D in those given vitamin D increased from 30.2 ng/ml to 61.1 ng/ml. Although in the case of the elderly (ages 67-86) there was no significantly improved balance as measured with the Sensory Organization Test (SOT), in the younger group (ages 52-66) researchers (after a post hoc analysis) found a significant improvement in the SOT. It can be assumed, based on the studies I will mention at the end of this part of the book, that the lack of such significant effects in the elderly is due to the fact that these people naturally need much more vitamin D to achieve the same levels as younger people.

Knekt, Paul et al. **"Serum vitamin D and the risk of Parkinson disease."** Archives of neurology 67 7 (2010): 808-11 .

3,173 men and women were included in the study. Of these, over 50 people developed Parkinson's disease over the 29-year follow-up period. The researchers commented on the study as follows: "This cohort study shows that low serum vitamin D level predicts an elevated risk of Parkinson's disease incidence. Individuals with a serum vitamin D concentration of at least 50 nmol/l had a 65% lower risk than those with values under 25 nmol/l after adjustment for several potential confounders (sex, age, marital status, education, alcohol consumption, smoking etc.) Despite the overall low vitamin D levels in the study population, a dose – response relationship was also found."

CHAPTER 6:
DEMENTIA AND ALZHEIMER'S DISEASE

Alzheimer's disease is a progressive brain disorder, which contributes to atrophy (a loss of brain cells over time). This disease is also the most common type of dementia, accounting for about 75% of all dementia cases. As the studies will show in a moment, it is also associated with vitamin D deficiency. This is because of the role of this vitamin in neurotrophy, neurotransmission, neuroprotection, and neuroplasticity.

Chai, Bingyan et al. "**Vitamin D deficiency as a risk factor for dementia and Alzheimer's disease: an updated meta-analysis.**" *BMC Neurology* 19 (2019): n. pag.

The aim of this meta-analysis was to examine the association between serum 25(OH)D deficiency and risk of dementia and Alzheimer's disease. The study included twelve prospective cohort studies and four cross-sectional studies. Scientists found that for vitamin D levels below 20 ng/ml, the risk of developing dementia increased by 32% and the risk of Alzheimer's disease by 34%. Moreover, the risk of developing dementia and Alzheimer's in people with 25(OH)D <10 ng/ml was 48% and 51% higher, respectively, compared to those with 10-20 ng/ml.

Littlejohns, Thomas J. et al. "**Vitamin D and the risk of dementia and Alzheimer disease**." Neurology 83 (2014): 920 - 928.

In another meta-analysis, the scientists came to similar

conclusions. 1,658 healthy people over the age of 65 were included in the study. After an average of 5.6 years, 171 participants developed dementia and 102 Alzheimer's disease. The researchers found that people with vitamin D deficiencies (10-20 ng/ml) had a 53% increased risk of developing dementia, while those severely deficient (<10 ng/ml) had as much as 125% compared to those with normal levels. For Alzheimer's disease, the risk increased by 70% for deficiency and 120% for severe deficiency. They indicated that the risk of developing dementia and Alzheimer's significantly increases to 50 nmol/l (20 ng/ml).

Miller, Joshua W. et al. **"Vitamin D Status and Rates of Cognitive Decline in a Multiethnic Cohort of Older Adults."** JAMA neurology 72 11 (2015): 1295-303 .

In this study, the researchers wanted to estimate the relationship between vitamin D levels and the rates of cognitive decline. 382 people with an average age of 75 and an average vitamin D level of 19 ng/ml were enrolled in this cohort study. They were people of different race/ethnicity and, interestingly, white people had this level higher than African American and Hispanic participants. What is important, however, moderately deficient (12-20 ng/ml) and severely deficient (<12 ng/ml) subjects had significantly greater annual decline in verbal memory compared to those with 25(OH)D levels of 20-50 ng/ml over a mean of 4.8 years. Thus, the conclusion from this study as well as from previous ones is that vitamin D supplementation is necessary in the elderly so that they can maintain their memory.

CHAPTER 7: AUTISM

Vitamin D plays a vital role in brain homeostasis, embryogenesis, neurodevelopment, brain's immunological modulation, neural differentiation and gene regulation, among others. This role can be especially important in autism. This disorder already affects at least 1 in 44 children in the U.S, of which boys are four times more likely to be diagnosed with autism than girls (prevalence of approx. 1 in 27). It has been estimated that the prevalence of autism has increased by almost 250% since 2000. Moreover, the predictions for the future are also not optimistic. However, there is also some good news. As various studies have shown, vitamin D may play a role in preventing the occurrence of autism in the offspring as well as significantly improving symptoms with supplementation.

Mostafa, G.A., & Al-Ayadhi, L. (2012). **Reduced serum concentrations of 25-hydroxy vitamin D in children with autism:** Relation to autoimmunity. Journal of Neuroinflammation, 9, 201 - 201.

In this publication, researchers tried to examine the relationship between vitamin D levels and anti-myelin-associated glycoprotein (anti-MAG) auto-antibodies (the level of these antibodies is usually significantly higher in autistic children than in healthy ones) in autistic children. They found that autistic children have significantly lower levels of vitamin D than healthy children. 48% of these children had vitamin D levels between 10-30 ng/ml. Moreover, as many as 40% of them had levels below 10 ng/ml. Increased levels of serum anti-MAG auto-antibodies were found in 70% of autistic children and were negatively correlated with vitamin D levels.

Chen, Jianzhang et al. "**Lower maternal serum 25(OH) D in first trimester associated with higher autism risk in Chinese offspring.**" Journal of psychosomatic research 89 (2016): 98-101

The authors of this publication compared the levels of vitamin D in mothers who gave birth to children who developed autism in the future and those whose children did not develop autism. The study included 68 autistic children and 68 healthy children. They used archived samples from the first trimester of pregnancy identified for every child. The results showed that "Mothers in autistic group had significantly lower maternal serum levels of 25(OH)D than in the typically-developing group, with 55.9% and 29.4% being vitamin D deficient, respectively (P<0.001). Levels of 25(OH)D increased with decreasing severity of ASD (Autism Spectrum Disorder) (...)". Thus, it was concluded from this study that the lower the maternal vitamin D level in the first trimester, the higher the risk of developing autism in offspring.

Saad, Khaled et al. "**Randomized controlled trial of vitamin D supplementation in children with autism spectrum disorder**." Journal of Child Psychology and Psychiatry 59 (2018): 20–29.

This double-blinded, randomized clinical trial was conducted on 85 ASD boys and 24 ASD girls aged 3-10 years. Patients were given vitamin D (300 IU/kg/day) or a placebo for 4 months. In contrast to the placebo group, the symptoms of autism improved significantly in these children in the vitamin D supplementation group within 4 months. The authors suggested that vitamin D may be recommended for children with autism for the safe and effective improvement of symptoms.

CHAPTER 8:
AMYOTROPHIC
LATERAL SCLEROSIS

Amyotrophic lateral sclerosis is a neurodegenerative disease that affects upper and lower motor neurons in the spinal cord and brain resulting in paralysis. The prevalence of this disease is about 6 cases per 100,000 people. Also in this case, studies suggest a positive effect of vitamin D.

Karam, Chafic et al. **"Vitamin D deficiency and its supplementation in patients with amyotrophic lateral sclerosis."** Journal of Clinical Neuroscience 20 (2013): 1550-1553.

Scientists have studied the impact of vitamin D on patients with amyotrophic lateral sclerosis (ALS). After measuring the vitamin D level of these patients, 81% of patients had a vitamin D level lower than 30 ng/mL and 43% had a vitamin D level lower than 20 ng/mL. Then twenty patients took 2000 IU of vitamin D daily for 9 months. Median 25(OH)D rose from 18.5 to 31.0 ng/mL at 6 months. After nine months, it was found that vitamin D had a positive effect on the Amyotrophic Lateral Sclerosis Functional Rating Scale (ALSFRS-R) score of these ALS patients.

Camu, William et al. **"Vitamin D confers protection to motoneurons and is a prognostic factor of amyotrophic lateral sclerosis."** Neurobiology of Aging 35 (2014): 1198-1205.

Other scientists have found a neuroprotective role for the biologically active form of vitamin D by, inter alia, preventing motoneurons from a Fas-induced death and potentiated effect of neurotrophic factors. They also mentioned about a four-time accelerated decline and reduced expectation of life due to severe vitamin D deficiency in patients with amyotrophic lateral sclerosis.

CHAPTER 9: MULTIPLE SCLEROSIS

Multiple sclerosis is a chronic and progressive demyelinating disease of the central nervous system, affecting mainly young adults. It is estimated that in the United States alone, nearly one million people suffer from multiple sclerosis. Damage to the brain and spinal cord by loss of the myelin sheaths of nerve fibers (demyelination) can lead to a wide variety of symptoms. These symptoms include vision problems (eye pain, decreased visual acuity and color vision impairment), muscle weakness, numbness and tingling, sensory disturbances, bladder problems, tremor, fatigue, and cognitive impairment. Vitamin D deficiency has been associated with an increased risk of developing multiple sclerosis, incidence of relapses and neurological disability. Studies have shown that vitamin D supplementation resulted in reduced magnetic resonance imaging (MRI) activity in relapsing-remitting multiple sclerosis patients. In addition, vitamin D has also been shown to be effective in reducing anti-EBNA-1 IgG levels. Based on several scientific publications, we will take a better look at these results and explain a little.

Rolf, Linda et al. **"Exploring the effect of vitamin D3 supplementation on the anti-EBV antibody response in relapsing-remitting multiple sclerosis."** Multiple Sclerosis (Houndmills, Basingstoke, England) 24 (2018): 1280 - 1287.

Infection with Epstein-Barr virus (EBV) dramatically increases the risk of developing multiple sclerosis (as some research shows up to 32 times). Approximately 90% of the population shows serologic signs of EBV infection. However, virtually all multiple sclerosis (MS) patients are EBV-seropositive (have antibodies to this virus in their blood). Anti-EBNA-1 immunoglobulin (igG) is an IgG antibody specific for the EBV EBNA protein. Higher anti-EBNA-1 igG levels are associated with an increased risk of MS. If that's already understood, let's move on to the study above. Participants were patients aged 18–55 years, treated with interferon-β1α, with relapsing-remitting multiple sclerosis. The division was made into the vitamin D group and the placebo group. In the vitamin D group, patients received 7,000 IU/day of vitamin D for 4 weeks and then 14,000 IU/day of vitamin D up to week 48. At the start of the study, the mean level of vitamin D in both groups together was 22 ng/ml and it did not change in the placebo group. In turn, in the group with vitamin D, the level of 25(OH)D increased to 92 ng/ml. As it turned out, after 48 weeks, there was a significant reduction of anti-EBNA-1 IgG levels in the group supplementing vitamin D. The effect of reducing anti-EBNA-1 IgG levels was not observed in the placebo group, however.

Munger, Kassandra L. et al. **"Vitamin D Status During Pregnancy and Risk of Multiple Sclerosis in Offspring of Women in the Finnish Maternity Cohort."** JAMA neurology 73 5 (2016): 515-9 .

Munger, Kassandra, et al, decided to investigate whether vitamin D levels in early pregnancy correlate with the risk of developing multiple sclerosis in the offspring. For this purpose they examined available serum samples from the pregnancy of mothers whose offspring developed multiple sclerosis. 70% of the data was from the first trimester of pregnancy. As it turned out, there is an almost two-fold risk of developing MS in the offspring of mothers with 25(OH)D concentrations below 12.02 ng/ml compared to people without vitamin D deficiency.

Ascherio, Alberto et al. **"Vitamin D as an early predictor of multiple sclerosis activity and progression."** JAMA neurology 71 3 (2014): 306-14 .

Initially, this study was designed to evaluate the impact of early versus delayed interferon beta-1b treatment in patients with CIS (clinically isolated syndrome, which may be the beginning of multiple sclerosis). Patients were measured for 25(OH)D levels. What the researchers found is significant: "Higher 25(OH)D levels predicted reduced MS activity and a slower rate of progression. A 50-nmol/L (20-ng/mL) increment in average serum 25(OH)D levels within the first 12 months predicted a 57% lower rate of new active lesions (P < .001), 57% lower relapse rate (P = .03), 25% lower yearly increase in T2 lesion volume (P < .001), and 0.41% lower yearly loss in brain volume (P = .07) from months 12 to 60. Similar associations were found between 25(OH)D measured up to 12 months and MS activity or progression from months 24 to 60."

Fitzgerald, Kathryn C. et al. **"Association of Vitamin D Levels With Multiple Sclerosis Activity and Progression in Patients Receiving Interferon Beta-1b."** JAMA neurology 72 12 (2015): 1458-65.

These researchers wanted to investigate the relationship between vitamin D and the course of multiple sclerosis in patients treated with interferon beta-1b. The study included 1,482 patients. In these patients, the 25(OH)D level was significantly inversely correlated with the number of new active lesions. Above 20 ng/ml was associated with 31% lower risk of new lesions. However, the lowest rate of new lesions was observed among patients with vitamin D levels greater than 40 ng/ml.

Munger KL, Zhang SM, O'Reilly E, Hernán MA, Olek MJ, Willett WC, Ascherio A. **Vitamin D intake and incidence of multiple sclerosis.** Neurology. 2004 Jan 13;62(1):60-5. doi: 10.1212/01.wnl.0000101723.79681.38. PMID: 14718698.

This large observational study included 187,563 women. During the follow-up, 173 cases of MS were confirmed. Women who took vitamin D had a 40% reduced risk of developing MS in the follow-up period between 1980 and 2001 compared to women who were not supplementing with vitamin D at that time. However, despite adjusting for MS factors such as age, smoking or latitude of residence at birth, it is important to remember that this is still only an observational study and some other factors may have been overlooked.

Hupperts, Raymond et al. **"Randomized trial of daily high-dose vitamin D3 in patients with RRMS receiving subcutaneous**

interferon β-1a." Neurology 93 (2019): e1906 - e1916.

SOLAR trial was one of the largest randomized, double-blind, placebo-controlled trials investigating treatment with SC interferon-β-1a with vitamin D or with placebo for 48 weeks in 229 MS patients. The vitamin D dose was 14007 IU/day. In those who supplemented with vitamin D, the number of lesions was significantly reduced by 32% compared to the group that did not receive vitamin D. There was also a trend towards lower ARR (annualized relapse rate) in patients treated with vitamin D. Were it not for the difficulty in recruiting patients, the duration of the study was shortened (from 96 weeks to 48 weeks) and the number of patients (from 348), perhaps the results would have been even better and more significant.

Camu, William et al. **"Cholecalciferol in relapsing-remitting MS: A randomized clinical trial (CHOLINE)."** Neurology® Neuroimmunology & Neuroinflammation 6 (2019): n. pag.

The latter study that I will mention in this section was also in patients treated with interferons. However, it lasted twice as long (96 weeks). During this time, patients received 100,000 IU of vitamin D (equivalent to approximately 7143 IU/day) or placebo every other week. In ninety patients who completed this study, vitamin D after 96 weeks contributed to a significant reduction in the annualized relapse rate, new hypointense T1-weighted lesions and progression of EDSS (Expanded Disability Status Scale - It is a way of measuring the extent to which someone is affected by multiple sclerosis by quantifying disability and changes).

For people suffering from an autoimmune disease (including multiple sclerosis), the Coimbra protocol is also worth considering. It is a method of treating autoimmune diseases with high doses of vitamin D in the range of 40,000 to 200,000 IU per day. The exact dosage is based on the parathyroid hormone levels. When we increase the dose of vitamin D, the level of this hormone should drop. The goal is to have parathyroid hormone levels as low as possible, but still within the normal range, as this is when vitamin D works most effectively. The person should be on a low calcium diet at this time. Importantly, therapy should be carried out with a knowledgeable doctor.

CHAPTER 10:
EPILEPSY

Epilepsy is one of the most common neurological disorders affecting almost 50 million people worldwide. The treatment mainly uses anti-seizure medications, which, however, may have serious side effects, such as cognitive impairment. Moreover, anti-seizure medications can reduce vitamin D levels. This is a particularly undesirable effect, as studies show the role of vitamin D in epilepsy. People with epilepsy have decreased levels of this vitamin (as a next study will show) and supplementation may provide some significant benefits.

Teagarden, Diane L. et al. **"Low vitamin D levels are common in patients with epilepsy."** Epilepsy Research 108 (2014): 1352-1356.

This study investigated vitamin D levels in epileptic patients who are taking antiepileptic drugs. 596 patients with an average age of 41 years were enrolled in the study. The mean vitamin D level was 22.5 ng/ml. Moreover, 45% of patients had 25(OH)D levels below 20 ng/ml. Scientists also distinguished the scale of vitamin D deficiency in people taking enzyme-inducing and non-enzyme-inducing antiepileptic drugs. In the first group, the deficiency affected 54% of people, and in the second, 37%.

Holló, András et al. **"Correction of vitamin D deficiency improves seizure control in epilepsy**: A pilot study." Epilepsy & Behavior 24 (2012): 131-133.

In this study, researchers wanted to investigate the effect of vitamin D on seizure frequency in 13 patients with epilepsy pharmacoresistant. Median serum 25(OH)D level at baseline in these patients was 11.8 ng/ml. The level below 30 ng/ml was found in 12 people. Level below 12 ng/ml in eight patients. Patients were given vitamin D in a dose of 40,000-200,000 IU to raise the 25(OH)D level at least above 30 ng/ml. Thereafter, patients received between 2,000 and 2,600 IU per day. After 90 days, there was a significant reduction of seizure numbers in 10 patients with a median reduction of 40%. In five patients, the reduction of seizure was even greater than 50%.

CHAPTER 11: CARDIOVASCULAR HEALTH

Although cardiovascular health is rarely associated with vitamin D, such a link does exist and is strong. We know that most body cells, including vascular smooth muscles, cardiomyocytes as well as endothelium of the vessels have vitamin D receptors. The protective effect of vitamin D may be related to the effect of this vitamin on vessel compliance, blood pressure, renin-angiotensin system (essential for regulation of blood pressure and fluid balance), glycemic control as well as parathyroid hormone level. The well-known anti-inflammatory properties of vitamin D may also be crucial. Hence, such a significant link has also been found by many studies between heart health and vitamin D. We will take a closer look at them.

Zhou, Ren et al. **"Lower Vitamin D Status Is Associated with an Increased Risk of Ischemic Stroke**: A Systematic Review and Meta-Analysis." Nutrients 10 (2018): n. pag.

These researchers wanted to investigate the link between vitamin D and stroke. To this end, they analyzed 19 studies; three case control studies and sixteen prospective studies, including the cohort study, and the randomized controlled trial. They found that lower vitamin D levels are associated with an increased risk of ischemic stroke. This risk may be higher by as much as 62%. Scientists suggested that this effect of vitamin D was probably due to its ability to prevent thrombosis and reduce inflammation.

Siadat ZD, Kiani K, Sadeghi M, Shariat AS, Farajzadegan Z, Kheirmand M. **Association of vitamin D deficiency and**

coronary artery disease with cardiovascular risk factors. J Res Med Sci. 2012;17(11):1052-1055.

In this study of 57 patients diagnosed with coronary artery disease upon coronary angiography and 62 individuals in the control group, the authors found a strong relationship between vitamin D and the risk of coronary artery disease. They achieved the following results: "Without adjustment, the chance of being affected by coronary artery disease in individuals with vitamin D deficiency is 3.49 times in comparison to those with normal vitamin D and after adjustment with risk factors, i.e., blood pressure, diabetes, smoking, obesity, physical activity and high blood cholesterol, this chance becomes 5.8 times."

Raed, Anas et al. **"Dose responses of vitamin D3 supplementation on arterial stiffness in overweight African Americans with vitamin D deficiency: A placebo controlled randomized trial."** PLoS ONE 12 (2017): n. pag.

Arterial stiffness is an independent risk factor for cardiovascular events. This study looked at the effect of different doses of vitamin D on arterial stiffness in 70 aged 13–45 years African Americans with vitamin D deficiency (serum 25(OH)D levels ≤ 20 ng/ml). The division into four groups has been made. The first group was given 18,000 IU (equivalent to 600 IU/day), the second group was given 60,000 IU (2,000 IU/day), the third group was given 120,000 IU (4,000 IU/day) of vitamin D and the fourth group was given a placebo. The study lasted sixteen weeks. After this time, arterial stiffness increased by 2% in the placebo group. In the group supplementing vitamin D in the amount of 600 IU/day, there was a slight stiffness of 0.1%. In contrast, in the group supplementing with 2,000 IU/day of vitamin D, there was a 2% improvement in arterial stiffness. However, even greater improvement was seen in the group supplementing with 4,000 IU/day. In this group there was a 10.4% reduction in arterial stiffness. There has therefore been a significant and rapid reduction in arterial stiffness as stated by one of the authors.

Alagacone, Shiran et al. **"The association between vitamin D deficiency and the risk of resistant hypertension."** Clinical and Experimental Hypertension 42 (2019): 177 - 180.

Alagacone, Verga, et al, investigated the prevalence of vitamin D deficiency in people with hypertension. They analyzed 2953 known hypertensive subjects surveyed by NHANES (National Health and Nutrition Examination Survey). Of these 2,953 people, 12% had resistant hypertension and 88% controlled hypertension. They found that the prevalence of 25(OH)D levels below 20 ng/ml in resistant hypertension and controlled hypertension groups was 61% and 46% respectively. This indicated that there is a statistically significant association between vitamin D deficiency and hypertension.

Other researchers have also come to similar conclusions. I will only mention them. There are studies showing that adult hypertension is 30% greater in the lowest quartile compared to the highest quartile of serum 25(OH)D. There are also those that suggest that the incident hypertension in men and women with levels below 15 ng/ml is over 6 times higher and over 2.5 times higher, respectively, compared to men and women with 25(OH)D levels above 30 ng/ml.

Pfeifer, Michael et al. "**Effects of a short-term vitamin D(3) and calcium supplementation on blood pressure and parathyroid hormone levels in elderly women.**" The Journal of clinical endocrinology and metabolism 86 4 (2001): 1633-7.

The increase in calcium supply can contribute to the reduction of both systolic and diastolic blood pressure. In this randomized, placebo-controlled study in 148 elderly women, researchers wanted to investigate the effects of supplementing calcium with vitamin D, as well as calcium alone, on blood pressure. Hence, one group got a small dose of vitamin D 800 IU/day along with 1,200 mg of calcium, while the other only got 1,200 mg of calcium. Meanwhile, the levels of 25(OH)D in people supplementing vitamin D increased by 72% (it's worth noting that people in this study started with levels below 20 ng/ml). While calcium contributed to a 4% decrease in blood pressure, it was 9.3% after 8 weeks for the vitamin D and calcium supplementation group. There was also a decrease in heart rate of 5.4%. However, it should be remembered that although in this case vitamin D supplementation with calcium gave positive results, this combination is not always beneficial. And what's more, with higher levels of vitamin D, additional calcium supplementation can do a lot of harm. More on that later.

CHAPTER 12:
DIABETES

Vitamin D also plays an important role in diabetes. Studies have shown that vitamin D deficiency impairs insulin synthesis and secretion in humans and in animal models of diabetes. A deficiency of this vitamin can significantly increase the risk of developing type 1 diabetes. A similar, though smaller, risk reduction was also seen in the case of type 2 diabetes. Furthermore, deficiency of this vitamin can contribute to the appearance of various diabetes complications, such as diabetic ulcers and diabetic retinopathy. Hence, it is so important to take care of the proper level of vitamin D in order not to develop diabetes, or, in case the disease is already there, to avoid unpleasant complications. Studies have shown that it is possible.

Hyppönen, Elina et al. **"Intake of vitamin D and risk of type 1 diabetes: a birth-cohort study."** The Lancet 358 (2001): 1500-1503.

This birth-cohort study included 12055 pregnant women from Northern Finland. 10,821 (91% of those surviving) children were followed-up at age 1 year. During the first year of life, data on the frequency and dose of vitamin D supplementation were also collected. From the group of children analyzed, 81 were diagnosed with diabetes type 1 during the study. As this analysis showed, with vitamin D supplementation, the risk of the frequency of type 1 diabetes (when adjusted for neonatal, anthropometric, and social characteristics) can be reduced by up to 88% compared to the case without supplementation. Furthermore, children who regularly took 2,000 IU of vitamin D had a 78% reduced risk of developing type 1 diabetes, compared with those children regularly receiving lower doses than the recommended amount of vitamin D.

Lucato, Paola et al. **"Low vitamin D levels increase the risk of type 2 diabetes in older adults**: A systematic review and meta-analysis." Maturitas 100 (2017): 8-15 .

This meta-analysis is about the relationship between vitamin D and the risk of type 2 diabetes in older adults. It is based on 9 studies and includes 28,258 older participants with a mean age of 67.7 years. Median follow-up period was 7.3 years and 2.863 participants (10.1%) developed diabetes during that time. As it turned out, people with the lowest vitamin D levels had from 17% to 31% greater risk of developing diabetes compared to those with the highest vitamin D levels.

Yammine, Kaissar et al. **"Is there an association between vitamin D and diabetic foot disease? A meta-analysis."** Wound Repair and Regeneration 28 (2019): n. pag.

Authors of another meta-analysis including 1,644 patients; 817 diabetic patients with foot ulcers and 827 patients having diabetes without foot complications investigated the relationship between vitamin D and the occurrence of diabetic foot. They stated that: "The quality of the included studies was found to be good to excellent. Diabetic foot complications are associated with significantly lower levels of vitamin D. Patients with diabetic ulcers or diabetic infection are at higher risk of bearing severe vitamin D deficiency. Knowing the beneficial effect of vitamin D on wound healing, it is likely that recognizing and supplementing with vitamin D could prevent or improve the outcomes of diabetic foot complications."

Luo, B., Gao, F., & Qin, L. (2017). **The Association between Vitamin D Deficiency and Diabetic Retinopathy in Type 2 Diabetes:** A Meta-Analysis of Observational Studies. Nutrients, 9.

Diabetic retinopathy is also a frequent complication of diabetes that contributes to damage to the blood vessels in the retina of the eye. In this meta-analysis of observational studies, scientists wanted to evaluate the relationship between vitamin D and retinopathy. To this end, they analyzed 15 studies with over 17,664 participants, of which 3,455 (19.6%) had been diagnosed with diabetic retinopathy. Vitamin D levels varied considerably between those affected with retinopathy, ranging from 9.2 to 32.6 ng/ml. Nevertheless, the result of this meta-analysis showed that people with diabetes and a vitamin D deficiency (25(OH)D levels below 20 ng/ml) have an increased risk of developing diabetic retinopathy.

Regarding the ailments associated with diabetes, it has also been proven that vitamin D may have a positive effect on wound healing in patients with diabetic foot ulcers. This is due to the influence on glycemic control. These patients have experienced beneficial effects on glucose homeostasis, LDL and HDL cholesterol. Other studies, in turn, indicated that vitamin D supplementation prevented the increase in plasma HbA1c (glycosylated hemoglobin - increased concentration of glycosylated hemoglobin is associated with an increased risk of developing diabetes late complications) and insulin resistance.

CHAPTER 13: CARDIO-METABOLIC HEALTH, OBESITY

After earlier chapters, it can be concluded that vitamin D has a positive effect on cardio-metabolic health. Now we will discuss some studies that have explored these aspects more generally. We will see that vitamin D may be related to hypertension, heart rate, serum fasting blood glucose, dyslipidemia and even waist circumference and obesity. Perhaps, therefore, this chapter will encourage those who are not particularly interested in their health, but their figure and appearance, to take vitamin D supplementation. We'll see.

Khayyatzadeh, Sayyed Saeed et al. **"High-dose vitamin D supplementation is associated with an improvement in several cardio-metabolic risk factors in adolescent girls: a nine-week follow-up study."** Annals of Clinical Biochemistry 55 (2018): 227 -235.

In this study, the authors examined the effects of vitamin D supplementation on cardio-metabolic risk factors in 988 healthy adolescent girls in Iran. At the start of the study, the mean vitamin D levels of these girls were 9.2 ng/ml and 90% of the girls had levels below 20 ng/ml. The participants were then administered 50,000 IU/week (equivalent to 7142 IU/ day) for 9 weeks. After this time, the average serum 25(OH)D level increased to 36 ng/ml and the levels below 20 ng were only observed in 16% of the girls. Vitamin D supplementation, however, resulted in significant reductions in diastolic blood pressure, heart rate, waist circumference, serum fasting blood glucose, total- and low-density lipoprotein-cholesterol.

Steinvil, Arie et al. **"Vitamin D deficiency prevalence and cardiovascular risk in Israel."** European Journal of Clinical Investigation 41 (2011): n. pag.

In this cross-sectional analysis, researchers investigated the relationship between vitamin D and cardiovascular (CVD) health. This is a large study of 34,874 individuals from Israel with a mean age of 55. The mean level of vitamin D in women was 22.7 ng/ml, while in men it was 23.2 ng/ml. Furthermore, vitamin D levels below 30 ng/ml were common in 77% of women and 79% of men. Subsequently two groups were formed for analysis. The first group included people with 25(OH)D levels below 15 ng/ml, whereas the second group consisted of people with vitamin D levels above 30 ng/ml. They found that those in the first group were more affected by hypertension, diabetes mellitus, dyslipidemia, obesity, and peripheral vascular disease. So that vitamin D is significantly correlated with cardiovascular health.

Vitamin D Supplements May Aid Weight Loss For Obese And Overweight People, Study Finds. Huffington Post, 2015. Accessed online May 21, http://www.huffingtonpost.co.uk/2015/05/08/vitamin-d-supplements-weight-loss-study_n_7239722.html

In another study, scientists wanted to investigate whether vitamin D could affect weight loss. 400 obese or overweight adults were put on the same balanced, low-calorie diet. These people were divided into three groups: those who took placebo, those who took 25,000 IU of vitamin D per month (equivalent to 833 IU/day), and those who took 100,000 IU of vitamin D per month (equivalent to 3333 IU/day). Those who did not supplement vitamin D lost an average of 1.2 kg, those who took 25,000 IU lost an average of 3.8 kg, while those who took 100,000 IU/month of vitamin D lost 5.4 kg. Regarding waist circumference: non-supplementers lost 3.21 cm (1.25 in), those who took 25,000 IU lost 4 cm (over 1.5 in) and those who took 100,000 IU over 5.48 cm (over 2 in). In conclusion, vitamin D turned out to be beneficial in the process of losing weight.

CHAPTER 14:
ASTHMA

Asthma is a chronic inflammation of the bronchial tubes that causes them to contract uncontrollably. Once we see the word "inflammation," we may immediately begin to think that vitamin D may help to some extent. And this is the case here. This is important because in the United States alone, about 25 million (1 in 13 people) suffer from this disease, and worldwide it is about 300 million people.

Sandhu MS, Casale TB. **The role of vitamin D in asthma**. Ann Allergy Asthma Immunol. 2010 Sep;105(3):191-9; quiz 200-2, 217. doi: 10.1016/j.anai.2010.01.013. Epub 2010 Mar 1. PMID: 20800785.

In the above publication, scientists outlined the different roles vitamin D plays in asthma. They conclude the results of their analysis this way: "We hypothesize that vitamin D supplementation may lead to improved asthma control by inhibiting the influx of inflammatory cytokines in the lung and increasing the secretion of interleukin 10 (that inhibits the production of proinflammatory cytokines) by T -regulatory cells and dendritic cells (that link innate and adaptive immunity)".

Yadav, M., & Mittal, K. (2013). **Effect of Vitamin D Supplementation on Moderate to Severe Bronchial Asthma**. The Indian Journal of Pediatrics, 81, 650-654.

The effectiveness of vitamin D was also verified by supplementation. One hundred asthmatic children were enrolled in this study. In addition to the usual treatment, one group of patients received 60,000 IU of vitamin D per month (equivalent to 2,000 IU per day), while the other group received a placebo. The study lasted 6 months. As it turned out, in the group that received vitamin D there was a significant reduction in exacerbations compared to placebo, a significant increase in PEFR (peak expiratory flow rate - test to measure air flowing out of the lungs) and a significant reduction in the need for steroids and emergency visits. In other words, there was a significant reduction in disease severity in those who supplemented with vitamin D.

Andújar-Espinosa, Rubén et al. **"Effect of vitamin D supplementation on asthma control in patients with vitamin D deficiency: the ACVID randomised clinical trial."** Thorax 76 (2020): 126 - 133.

This study is similar to the previous one. It is a randomized, triple-blind, placebo-controlled, parallel-group study in adult asthma patients but having 25(OH)D levels below 30 ng/ml. For standard treatment, one group received 16,000 IU of vitamin D (equivalent to about 2,300 IU/day), while the other group received a placebo. The study period was 6 months. A statistically significant clinical improvement was observed in the group who supplemented vitamin D compared to the control group (as measured using asthma control test). In addition, the quality of life in the supplementation group improved significantly.

CHAPTER 15:
CYSTIC FIBROSIS

About 85-90% of people with cystic fibrosis suffer from insufficient pancreas and impaired fat absorption. For this reason, it is estimated that up to 90% of people with this disease are deficient in vitamin D. This, in turn, further aggravates the health situation. Additional supplementation could prove very beneficial. Vitamin D may induce expression of cathelicidin by macrophages and monocytes. Cathelicidin eliminates pathogenic microbes and modulates host immune responses. In addition, vitamin D down regulates pro-inflammatory cytokines in macrophages as well as reduces inflammation in the airway. This is especially important because people with cystic fibrosis are at high risk of lung infections and are often hospitalized for this reason. However, infections aren't the only problem for people with cystic fibrosis.

Wolfenden, Linda L. et al. "**Vitamin D and bone health in adults with cystic fibrosis.**" Clinical Endocrinology 69 (2008): n. pag.

In this study, researchers tried to assess the prevalence of vitamin D insufficiency and its impact on bone and respiratory health in adults with cystic fibrosis (CF). For this purpose, 185 adults with CF with a mean age of 29 were enrolled in the study. As it turned out, over 76% of patients had 25(OH)D levels below 30 ng/ml. The mean level in these patients was about 23 ng/ml. There was also a slight, but significant, positive association between serum 25(OH)D and FEV(1) (Forced expiratory volume in one second - the volume of air exhaled in the first second during forced exhalation). Moreover, vertebral fractures were detected in as many as 27% of patients, which may be related to vitamin D deficiency in these patients.

The matter concerning bones is important in this case because the prevalence of osteopenia, osteoporosis vertebral and non-vertebra fractures may range from a dozen to several dozen percent in the group of people with CF (as research usually shows 15-40% depending on the type of bone problem).

Grossmann, Ruth E. et al. "**Pilot study of vitamin D supplementation in adults with cystic fibrosis pulmonary exacerbation.**" *Dermato-endocrinology* 4 (2012): 191 - 197.

There are also a few studies in which people with cystic fibrosis were given vitamin D. In this randomized controlled double blind placebo controlled trial, researchers investigated the effects of vitamin D on pulmonary exacerbation in patients with cystic fibrosis. Thirty CF patients hospitalized for pulmonary exacerbation were randomized to receive a single oral dose of 250,000 IU of vitamin D or placebo. Mean serum 25(OH)D in these vitamin D supplementation patients increased from 30.6 ng/ml to 58.1 ng/ml at one week and to 36.7 ng/ml by 12 weeks. Patients who received 250000 IU of vitamin D had better antibiotic therapy-free days, hospital-free days and one year survival compared to the placebo group. Inflammatory markers such as interleukin-6 or tumor necrosis factor-α (TNF-α) were also significantly reduced.

CHAPTER 16:
PSORIASIS

Now is a good time to discuss the role of vitamin D in today's very common skin conditions such as psoriasis, eczema and acne. This role is huge and very broad. Vitamin D is responsible for the regulation of keratinocyte (primary cell type of the epidermis) apoptosis, promotion of keratinocyte differentiation and inhibition of keratinocyte proliferation. Vitamin D also plays an important immunomodulatory role and contributes to maintaining the proper epidermal barrier. In a moment I will show you what it means in practice.

Mahtani, Renu, and Pradeep M. Nair. **"Daily oral vitamin D3 without concomitant therapy in the management of psoriasis: A case series."** Clinical Immunology Communications, vol. 2, 2022, pp. 17-22, https://doi.org/10.1016/j.clicom.2022.01.001.

At the very beginning, I would like to refer to an exceptional scientific publication that appeared in 2022. This is a report of 6 cases of treating psoriasis with vitamin D. Doses ranged from 30,000 IU to 60,000 IU per day over a period of 2 to 6 months and then followed by lower daily maintenance dose. These doses were adjusted based on parathyroid hormone levels as well as ionized calcium levels to prevent hypercalcemia. Monitoring parathyroid hormone levels can be used as a good indicator to estimate the optimal therapeutic doses of vitamin D. Low vitamin D levels result in higher parathyroid hormone levels. In the case of supplementation with vitamin D, the level of parathyroid hormone should drop. I have already mentioned in a chapter on multiple sclerosis that vitamin D is most effective when the parathyroid hormone levels are low but still within the normal range. In the case of vitamin D resistance, however, when the decrease in PTH is disturbed, then an increased dose of vitamin D is able to overcome this resistance and bring better results. It is important to remember that such resistance is more common in people with autoimmune diseases. And now let's move on to these cases.

Case 1. A woman aged 58 suffered from psoriasis for 30 years and severely from 6 years. She had intense itching, and erythematous scaly plaques on the body. Her baseline 25(OH)D level was 11 ng/ml and a PTH value of 65 pg/ml. The woman got 600,000 IU at the beginning and then 30,000 IU daily for 2 months. Due to the clinical improvement, the dose was reduced to 25,000 IU per day. The PTH levels also reduced to 37.5 pg/ml. After three months, the disease was completely controlled and without itching. The woman is now taking a maintenance dose of 20,000 IU per day. Her PTH and ionized calcium levels are well in range.

Case 2. Woman at 63 years old with itching and thick scaly eruptions. Her vitamin D was 45 ng/ml and her PTH level was 37.5 pg/ml at the beginning. The woman was getting 30,000 IU/day of vitamin D for 3 months. Her ionized calcium levels remained within the normal range at 1.25 ml/dl. After three months, the disease was completely controlled. The woman received the same maintenance dose as in the first case and by the end of the follow-up year she had no relapse.

Case 3. A 55-year-old woman has been struggling with psoriasis for 14 years, with severity in the last 2. Her vitamin D level was 9.44 ng/ml and PTH levels was 52.2 pg/mL. The woman was given a single dose of 600,000 IU then took 30,000 IU for 2 months. Due to the lack of significant improvement and still not the lowest PTH level (35.38 pg/mL after 2 months), the dose increased to 45,000 IU per day from the third month. Disease control was achieved by the end of the 6th month. The maintenance dose was progressively reduced to 15,000 IU now.

Case 4. A 37-year-old man had psoriasis for 8 years with worsening with some symptoms from 3 years. His vitamin D level was relatively high (61 ng/ml) and his PTH level was 24 pg/ml. The man was getting 30,000 IU a day for two months. Due to clinical improvement, this dose was reduced to 20,000 IU after 3 months. Complete control was achieved by the end of the 4th month. Currently, the maintenance dose is 15,000 IU.

Case 5. A 48-year-old woman with psoriasis had a vitamin D level of 21 ng/mL and a high PTH level of 113 pg/mL. Because of 90 percent subsidence in the progression of disease, her daily dose was reduced from 30,000 IU to 15,000 IU after 2 months. Until complete remission (i.e. by the end of the 4th month), the dose was reduced to 10,000 IU and has remained so until now.

Case 6. The last case is a 55-year-old woman with 8-year-long psoriasis with severe itching and erythrodermic lesions. Her 25(OH)D was 39 ng/ml and PTH levels at 26 pg/mL. Initially, this woman was getting 30,000 IU per day, but after a week, due to her BMI, the dose was increased to 40,000 IU per day. The dose was then increased to 50,000 IU after one month. As PTH levels dropped slightly, the authors concluded that this was associated with high resistance to this vitamin. Therefore, from the third month onwards, the dose was increased to 60,000 IU/day. Then this treatment was combined with a diet very low in calcium. After one month of such doses, PTH levels had dropped to 19 pg/ml and the ionized calcium levels were within the normal range. After another month, vitamin D was reduced at a rate of 10,000 IU per month. Complete control of the disease was achieved at month 8. The woman is now on a maintenance dose of 40,000 IU daily without hypercalcemia.

To summarize this briefly. Vitamin D given in high doses (often 20 times those commonly recommended and often used in other clinical studies) has been shown to be extremely effective in psoriasis without any side effects. Despite the fact that this study was small, we can assume that the introduction of this type of therapy could bring much better results than the standard treatment. What's more, knowing that vitamin D is also strongly associated with other diseases, we can assume that also in the case of these other diseases, this type of therapy, i.e. with high doses of vitamin D, could bring much better results.

Gisondi, Paolo et al. **"Vitamin D status in patients with chronic plaque psoriasis."** British Journal of Dermatology 166 (2012): n. pag.

In this study, the authors compared vitamin D levels in people with chronic plaque psoriasis, rheumatoid arthritis, and healthy people. A cross-sectional study was conducted over 1 year.

145 patients with chronic plaque psoriasis, 112 patients with rheumatoid arthritis and 141 healthy controls participated in it. The mean levels of vitamin D in these subjects were 20.7 ng/ml, 24ng/ml and 37 ng/ml respectively. In other words, 57.8% of patients with psoriasis had vitamin D levels below 20 ng/ml, whereas for healthy people it was 29.7%. Moreover, in winter, the prevalence of levels below 20 ng/ml in people with psoriasis was 80.9%. This proved that vitamin D deficiency is very common in people with this disease.

CHAPTER 17:
ECZEMA

Eczema (atopic dermatitis) is a condition similar to psoriasis. It is characterized by itchy and dry skin as well as the appearance of a rash inside the elbows, behind the knees, on the hands, face and feet. As with psoriasis, eczema patients have decreased levels of vitamin D, and supplementation with this vitamin helps to reduce symptoms. Several studies proved this.

El Taieb, Moustafa A. et al. "**Assessment of Serum 25-Hydroxyvitamin D Levels in Children with Atopic Dermatitis: Correlation With SCORAD Index.**" Dermatitis 24 (2013): 296–301.

The authors of this publication compared the mean levels of vitamin D in healthy children and those suffering from atopic dermatitis (AD). In addition, they compared vitamin D levels for mild, moderate, and severe stages of this disease in these 2-12 year olds. The mean result in the control group was significantly higher than in the group of children with AD (28.9 ng/ml vs 5.4 ng/ml). Moreover, the levels of 25(OH)D in children with mild AD (14.6 ng/ml) were significantly higher than in those with moderate AD (5.5 ng/ml) and severe AD (0.3 ng/ml). This study therefore revealed very serious vitamin D deficiencies that endanger the health and life of these children. If such a level of 25(OH)D shows up after the test, whether for children or adults, according to what science says, it should be corrected immediately.

Amestejani, Morteza et al. "**Vitamin D supplementation in the treatment of atopic dermatitis: a clinical trial study.**" Journal of drugs in dermatology : JDD 11 3 (2012): 327-30 .

For this randomized, double-blind, placebo-controlled trial

study, 60 people with atopic dermatitis were enrolled. These people were divided into two groups that received either 1,600 IU of vitamin D per day or a placebo for 60 days. In the group supplementing vitamin D, there was a significant improvement in the severity of the disease based on SCORAD (Scoring Atopic Dermatitis) and TIS (Three Item Severity score) in patients with mild, moderate and severe AD.

In addition, vitamin D supplementation also turns out to be effective in an adjuvant treatment in the case of severe atopic dermatitis along with such agents as e.g. popular hydrocortisone creams.

Camargo, Carlos A. et al. "**Randomized trial of vitamin D supplementation for winter-related atopic dermatitis in children.**" The Journal of allergy and clinical immunology 134 4 (2014): 831-835.e1 .

107 children with mean age of 9 years with winter-related atopic dermatitis participated in another randomized, double-blind, placebo-controlled trial. The children were given 1,000 IU of vitamin D per day or a placebo for one month. As it turned out, vitamin D supplementation for 1 month produced a clinically and statistically significant improvement in EASI (Eczema Area and Severity Index) score in these children. So the authors concluded: "Vitamin D supplementation improved winter-related AD among Mongolian children, a population likely to have vitamin D deficiency in winter."

CHAPTER 18: ACNE

Acne is one of the most common skin conditions worldwide. In the United States alone, it affects up to 50 million Americans annually. In addition, approximately 85% of people between the ages of 12 and 24 have at least minor acne. This often leads to emotional problems, including mood disorders, sleep problems or obsession with their own appearance. Vitamin D may prove beneficial. Vitamin D works in several ways here. It reduces the expression of IL17, elevated levels of which are found in people with acne. It reduces the expression of inflammatory cytokines such as interleukin IL-6, IL-8, and matrix metalloproteinase 9. Another mechanism of action may also be the inducing antimicrobial peptides such as LL-37 in human sebocytes. Beyond theory, scientists have also shown these helpful effects of vitamin D in practice.

Wang, Meng et al. **"Vitamin D status and efficacy of vitamin D supplementation in acne patients: A systematic review and meta-analysis."** Journal of Cosmetic Dermatology 20 (2021): n. pag.

The authors of this systematic review and meta-analysis wanted to investigate the relationship between vitamin D and acne vulgaris. Both the studies comparing 25(OH)D levels and case-controls or randomized controlled trials indicated the effectiveness of vitamin D in this ailment. Researchers also calculated, based on many studies, that the difference in vitamin D levels between healthy and acne-affected people is 7.7 ng/ml on average.

Ahmed Mohamed, Amal et al. **"The impact of active vitamin D administration on the clinical outcomes of acne vulgaris."** Journal of Dermatological Treatment 32 (2019): 756 - 761.

100 healthy people and 100 people with acne participated in this

study. Acne patients were divided into two groups. One group received 0.25 μg of alfacalcidol (It is a vitamin D derivative which can undergo hydroxylation in the liver to 1,25(OH)2D - active form) daily and the other group received placebo for three months. As it turned out, the level of the 25(OH)D metabolite in people with acne was significantly lower than in the group of healthy people before the intervention. Moreover, as a result of vitamin D supplementation, there was a favorable and significant reduction in the median serum level of IL6 and pro-inflammatory TNFα as compared to placebo and the initial levels.

CHAPTER 19: CHRONIC URTICARIA

Vitamin D, due to its immunoregulatory and anti-inflammatory properties, may prove to be effective in the treatment of a common allergic skin condition, which is chronic urticaria.

Rorie A, Goldner WS, Lyden E, Poole JA. **Beneficial role for supplemental vitamin D3 treatment in chronic urticaria: a randomized study.** Ann Allergy Asthma Immunol. 2014 Apr;112(4):376-82. doi: 10.1016/j.anai.2014.01.010. Epub 2014 Feb 5. PMID: 24507460.

Rorie, Goldner, et al, examined the effects of vitamin D on chronic urticaria. Forty-two subjects with chronic urticaria participated in this prospective, double-blinded, single-center study. One group received 4,000 IU daily of vitamin D and the other 600 IU for 12 weeks. In addition, all subjects were given triple-drug therapy (cetirizine, ranitidine, and montelukast). The Urticaria Symptom Severity (USS) score decreased by 33% after one week due to triple-drug therapy. In the higher dose group (there was no such effect at the lower dose), the USS score decreased further by 40% by week 12. There was a trend toward lower total USS scores at week 12 in the 4000 IU dose group versus the 600 IU dose group associated with significantly reduced distribution on the body and frequency of hives. Additionally, beneficial trends for sleep quality and pruritus scores appeared in the group supplementing higher doses of vitamin D.

CHAPTER 20:
WOUND HEALING

Vitamin D is also essential in the process of wound healing when the skin gets injured. This is due to a fact that I have already mentioned, namely that vitamin D promotes the production of cathelicidin, an antimicrobial peptide, which prevents wound infections and thus shortens the wound healing time.

Smith, K., & Hewlings, S.J. (2020). **Correlation between vitamin D levels and hard-to-heal wounds: a systematic review.** Journal of wound care, 29 Sup7, S24-S30 .

In this systematic review, researchers investigated this relationship between vitamin D and wound healing. For this task, they analyzed 10 studies, involving 2,359 participants, which met the inclusion criteria. They found a strong correlation between the low 25(OH)D level and the presence of three types of hard-to-heal wounds (primary, secondary, and tertiary). Moreover, they also pointed to the existence of a rationale for using vitamin D for the treatment of hard-to-heal wounds.

CHAPTER 21: OSTEOARTHRITIS

Osteoarthritis is a disease characterized by joint pain, joint space narrowing, osteophyte formation, and cartilage damage. It is estimated that 13% of women and 10% of men over the age of 60 have symptomatic knee osteoarthritis. Worse still, nearly half of them will have a total knee replacement. The way vitamin D works in this disease is not fully known. Vitamin D is presumed to act both directly, as there are vitamin D receptors on damaged cartilage, and indirectly, through the endocrine system. Despite the uncertainty, vitamin D supplementation has been shown to be effective in many studies.

Gao, Xu-Ren et al. **"The effect of vitamin D supplementation on knee osteoarthritis: A meta-analysis of randomized controlled trials."** International journal of surgery 46 (2017): 14-20 .

The above meta-analysis is based on four studies conducted in the US, UK, China and India. The daily dose of vitamin D varied from 800 IU to 60,000 IU between studies. The researchers found that the arthritic symptoms were significantly improved in the group that supplemented with vitamin D. Importantly, however, to obtain the desired effect, this dose had to be higher than 2,000 IU per day.

CHAPTER 22:
RHEUMATOID
ARTHRITIS

Rheumatoid arthritis, unlike osteoarthritis, which is primarily a degenerative joint disorder, has an autoimmune origin. We already know that the first thing that should be associated with an autoimmune disease is vitamin D or rather lack of it. Vitamin D controls the innate and adaptive immune systems. Vitamin D is an important regulator of various genes involved in the immune system. And vitamin D prevents the occurrence and development of rheumatoid arthritis, mainly through inhibiting cytokine levels. Also, studies have shown an inverse relationship between this disease and vitamin D levels. We will briefly look at them.

Lee, Y.H., & Bae, S.-. (2016). **Vitamin D level in rheumatoid arthritis and its correlation with the disease activity: a meta-analysis**. Clinical and experimental rheumatology, 34 5, 827-833 .

The meta-analysis was based on 15 studies involving 1,143 patients with rheumatoid arthritis. The scientists concluded the results: "Our meta-analysis demonstrates that serum vitamin D level is significantly low in patients with RA (rheumatoid arthriti), vitamin D deficiency is prevalent in RA patients compared to controls (55.2% vs. 33.2%), and the vitamin D level correlates inversely with RA activity. Our meta-analysis suggests that the vitamin D level is associated with susceptibility to RA and RA activity."

Song, Gwan Gyu et al. **"Association between vitamin D intake and the risk of rheumatoid arthritis: a meta-analysis."** Clinical

Rheumatology 31 (2012): 1733-1739.

Another meta-analysis was based on three cohort studies including 215,757 participants and eight studies involving 2,885 rheumatoid arthritis (RA) patients and 1,084 controls. Scientists found a significant association between total vitamin D intake and RA incidence. People in the highest group for total vitamin D intake were found to have a over 24% lower risk of developing rheumatoid arthritis than those people in the lowest group.

Tabatabaeizadeh, Seyed-Amir et al. **"High Dose Supplementation of Vitamin D Affects Measures of Systemic Inflammation: Reductions in High Sensitivity C-Reactive Protein Level and Neutrophil to Lymphocyte Ratio (NLR) Distribution."** Journal of Cellular Biochemistry 118 (2017): n. pag.

Both the neutrophil count and the C-Reactive Protein (CRP) level are usually elevated in people with rheumatoid arthritis. The above study was designed to investigate the effect of vitamin D on these measures of inflammation. 580 adolescent girls took part in this study. They took 50,000 IU of vitamin D at weekly intervals for 9 weeks (equivalent to about 7,100 IU per day) After this time, researchers observed a significant reduction in neutrophil count and CRP level after the vitamin D supplementation.

CHAPTER 23:
ANEMIA

Anemia is usually associated by doctors and ordinary people with a deficiency of iron, folic acid or vitamin B12. However, it turns out that vitamin D deficiency may also contribute to this ailment. Several studies have found such a link.

Nur-Eke, R., & Özen, M. (2020). **The Relationship between Vitamin D Levels and Iron Deficiency and Anemia in Adults Applied for Periodic Medical Examination.** Clinical laboratory, 66 6.

Due to this evidence from other studies, Nur-Eke and Özen decided to investigate it more accurately. The authors included over 9,590 adults (aged 18-64) in the analysis, of which 1,470 were anemic patients. In addition, these patients were classified into three groups as iron deficiency, iron deficiency anemia, and anemia. Iron, hemoglobin (Hgb), and ferritin levels were found to be significantly lower in the vitamin D deficient group than in those without. The level of 25(OH)D in people with anemia was 14% lower than in healthy people, in people with iron deficiency it was 12% and in people with iron deficiency anemia it was almost 18%. As the authors concluded: "The findings of this large study population, who live in a Mediterranean city which is sunny for 300 days of the year, indicate that 25(OH)D deficiency is significantly associated with iron deficiency and/or anemia."

CHAPTER 24:
CROHN'S DISEASE

Crohn's disease is a chronic autoimmune inflammatory disease. The inflammatory process caused by this disease affects the gastrointestinal wall and may affect its various areas, although most often it takes place in the final section of the ileum. The most common symptoms include diarrhea, abdominal pain, weight loss, and malnutrition-related anemia. Unfortunately, medicine is almost helpless in this case, it is not talking about curing the patients, but only reducing the symptoms. Complete remissions are very rare. However, there are also reports of cures of this supposedly incurable disease. Doctors who achieve these results also use vitamin D in higher doses for treatment. While there is no study that examines this phenomenon using high doses of vitamin D, it turns out there are studies that show vitamin D efficacy against this disease even at relatively low doses and 25(OH)D levels.

Yang, Linlin et al. **"Therapeutic Effect of Vitamin D Supplementation in a Pilot Study of Crohn's Patients."** Clinical and Translational Gastroenterology 4 (2013): n. pag.

In this study, researchers raised vitamin D levels above 40 ng/ml in patients with mild-to-moderate Crohn's disease and evaluated the influence of this vitamin on health condition. Patients were given vitamin D at a dose of 1000 IU/day and after 2 weeks, the dose was escalated incrementally until patients' serum concentrations reached 40 ng/ml 25(OH)D or they were taking 5,000 IU/day. 78% of patients required a dose of 5,000 IU/day. Scientists found that vitamin D supplementation significantly reduced the unadjusted mean Crohn's disease activity index (CDAI) scores by 112 points from 230 to 118. Furthermore, Quality-of-life scores also improved.

CHAPTER 25:
THYROID HEALTH

While I will look at the health of the thyroid gland in more detail in the iodine part of this book, it turns out that vitamin D also plays a role in thyroid disease. The exact mechanisms by which vitamin D works in this regard have not been investigated yet, but a significant relationship between this vitamin and thyroid disease has been already found by many studies.

Taheriniya, Sorour et al. **"Vitamin D and thyroid disorders: a systematic review and Meta-analysis of observational studies."** BMC Endocrine Disorders 21 (2021): n. pag.

This meta-analysis from 2021 is the result of an analysis of 35 observational studies published between 1980 and 2018 regarding thyroid diseases. Vitamin D was found to be significantly associated with hypothyroidism, autoimmune thyroid diseases and Hashimoto's thyroiditis. Moreover, 25(OH)D levels were significantly lower in people over 40 years old with Graves' disease.

CHAPTER 26:
FIBROMYALGIA

Fibromyalgia is a disorder characterized by extensive musculoskeletal pain accompanied by chronic fatigue, sleep disturbances, and psychopathological symptoms. There are several studies that show that people with this condition are severely deficient in vitamin D, and supplementation helps reduce symptoms. Importantly, they also indicate that the levels of vitamin D that provide relief must often be higher than those found on average in healthy people (over 50 ng/ml).

Bhatty, Shaheen et al. "**Vitamin D deficiency in fibromyalgia.**" JPMA. The Journal of the Pakistan Medical Association 60 11 (2010): 949-51.

Bhatty, Shaikh, et al, wanted to investigate vitamin D levels in people with fibromyalgia. For this reason, 40 women with an average age of 38 were enrolled in the study. 80% of the subjects had a 25(OH)D level below 20 ng/ml and the mean level was 15.8 ng/ml. On the other hand, 20% of people had levels between 21-29 ng/ml. In this group, the mean level of 25(OH)D was 23.6 ng/ml. This study therefore proved that vitamin D deficiencies are very common in people with fibromyalgia.

de Carvalho, Jozélio Freire et al. "**Vitamin D Supplementation Seems to Improve Fibromyalgia Symptoms: Preliminary Results.**" The Israel Medical Association journal : IMAJ 20 6 (2018): 379-381.

In another study, researchers analyzed the effect of vitamin D supplementation on fibromyalgia symptoms. Eleven female patients with fibromyalgia diagnosis and 25(OH)D values ≤ 30 ng/ml were enrolled. Then, they received 50,000 IU per week (equivalent to 7142 IU/day) for a period of three months. These people's 25(OH)D levels increased from 18.3 ng/ml to 33.8 ng/ml after these three months. Eight patients (72%) experienced very significant improvement in symptoms. Moreover, after three months, a trend for reduction of the number of tender points (areas where patients may experience pain when they are pressed) was observed.

Mirzaei, Alireza et al. **"Effects of vitamin D optimization on quality of life of patients with fibromyalgia: A randomized controlled trial."** Medical Journal of the Islamic Republic of Iran 32 (2018): 29 - 29.

Another randomized controlled trial involved 74 FMS patients with hypovitaminosis D. Among them, 64 patients were identified with vitamin D < 20 ng/ml and 10 with vitamin D levels 20.1-29 ng/ml. Two groups were given 25 mg of Trazodone (it's a popular antidepressant, often recommended to these patients to improve sleep quality). In addition, one group received 50,000 IU of vitamin D a week, as in the previous study, and the other group received a placebo. It turned out that the combination of Trazodone with vitamin D resulted in significant improvement of SF-36 (Short Form Health Survey) scores compared to Trazodone therapy only. Scientists concluded it like this: "This study suggests that vitamin D supplementation has significant therapeutic benefits in the management of FMS, especially in pain reduction of patients with fibromyalgia. According to our results, a combination of vitamin D supplements and a conventional antidepressant, when given to vitamin D-deficient fibromyalgia patients, could significantly improve both physical and psychological symptoms "

Matthana, M.H. (2011). **The relation between vitamin D deficiency and fibromyalgia syndrome in women**. Saudi medical journal, 32 9, 925-9 .

Moving on to the last study in this chapter. 100 women suffering from fibromyalgia syndrome participated in this prospective cohort study. They were given 50,000 IU per week of ergocalciferol (vitamin D2) until their serum 25(OH)D levels exceeded 50 ng/ml. The results showed that 42 of the 61 vitamin

D-deficient fibromyalgia patients had significantly improved health status if their 25(OH)D levels had risen above 30 ng/ml. Moreover, the improvement was even more significant if the blood vitamin D levels exceeded 50 ng/ml.

CHAPTER 27: PCOS

Polycystic ovary syndrome (PCOS) is one of the most common endocrine disorders of reproductive age women. This ailment affects 6-12% of women, although some data mention up to 20%. As various studies have shown, vitamin D deficiencies are common in people with PCOS. In addition, the correction of these deficiencies or increasing the levels of 25(OH)D may have several benefits for patients. I will explain them briefly:

1. PCOS negatively affects fertility. Women who are deficient in vitamin D may have difficulty producing mature eggs, which is essential for pregnancy. Deficiencies of this vitamin may affect the poor functioning of the uterus. Furthermore, there are also studies showing that vitamin D supplementation can regulate the course of the menstrual cycle.

2. PCOS is associated with anxiety (50% of women with PCOS) and depression (almost 30% of women). Vitamin D, in turn, plays a very important role in depression. Nevertheless, more details I will provide later in the chapter about depression.

3. Metabolic syndrome affects one in three women with PCOS. Vitamin D, however, as we already know, has a positive effect on diabetes and the circulatory system. Hence, supplementation can help improve the condition.

CHAPTER 28:
ENDOMETRIOSIS

Endometriosis is a disease involving the presence of endometrial cells outside their normal location, which is the uterine cavity. They may then be found in the peritoneal cavity, ovaries and fallopian tubes, the cervix and even the urinary bladder. A woman with endometriosis suffers from severe abdominal pain and painful periods. Other symptoms associated with this disease also include painful urination, intestinal problems, chronic fatigue, mood swings and infertility. The disease is commonly considered incurable and treatments mainly include hormone medicines, contraceptives, painkillers, and surgery. Actually studies and medical practice show that also other remedies can help significantly and, moreover, do not cause any side effects. Vitamin D is one of them. Studies have indicated not only that level of vitamin D is reduced in women with endometriosis, but also that this vitamin can alleviate symptoms.

Ciavattini, Andrea et al. **"Ovarian endometriosis and vitamin D serum levels**." Gynecological Endocrinology 33 (2017): 164 - 167.

The aim of this study was to evaluate the correlation between the level of 25(OH)D in women with ovarian endometriosis and the dimensions of ovarian endometriomas. The study included 49 women with a mean vitamin D level of 22 ng/ml, of which 42 of them (85.7%) were classified as having hypovitaminosis D. In people with vitamin D deficiency, the mean diameter of ovarian endometriomas was 40.2 mm, whereas in those without deficiency, 26.7 mm. Interestingly, researchers found a significant linear correlation between 25(OH)D serum level and the diameter of ovarian endometriomas.

Mehdizadehkashi, Abolfazl et al. **"The effect of vitamin D**

supplementation on clinical symptoms and metabolic profiles in patients with endometriosis." Gynecological Endocrinology 37 (2021): 640 - 645.

In this randomized, double-blind, placebo-controlled trial, scientists examined the effect of vitamin D on clinical symptoms and metabolic profiles in patients with endometriosis. The study was conducted on 60 patients aged 18-40 years old with endometriosis. One group received 50,000 IU (equivalent to approximately 3,570 IU/day) of vitamin D every two weeks for 12 weeks, while the other group was given a placebo. As it turned out, vitamin D supplementation significantly decreased pelvic pain and total- / HDL-cholesterol ratio compared with placebo. Furthermore, vitamin D supplementation resulted in a significant reduction in high-sensitivity C-reactive protein and significant increase in total antioxidant capacity.

CHAPTER 29:
BENIGN PROSTATIC HYPERPLASIA

Benign prostatic hyperplasia is caused by excessive growth of both epithelial and stromal cells of the prostate. It is a very common condition. About 50% of all men over the age of 50 will have this disease. After the age of 80, an enlarged prostate may affect up to 90% of men. As with many other ailments, vitamin D may prove beneficial here too. This is due to both the strong anti-inflammatory properties of this vitamin, which I have already mentioned many times, and the influence on the activity of various genes that may contribute to the development of this disease.

Zendehdel, Abolfazl et al. **"The effect of vitamin D supplementation on the progression of benign prostatic hyperplasia**: A randomized controlled trial." Clinical nutrition (2020): n. pag.

This study was conducted on 108 participants over 50 years of age. The patients were divided into two groups. One group got 50,000 IU of vitamin D every two weeks for six months, the other group got a placebo. Vitamin D improved benign prostatic hyperplasia symptoms, reduced prostate volume and prostate-specific antigen (PSA) levels (that are often elevated in this ailment).

Therefore, on the basis of this study only, one should conclude that every older man should take vitamin D supplementation, which may either protect him from benign prostatic hyperplasia or reduce his symptoms once the condition is present. It is a message to all daughters, sons, granddaughters and grandsons.

CHAPTER 30: ERECTILE DYSFUNCTION

The overall prevalence of erectile dysfunction has been estimated at 18% to 47% in the US, and this prevalence increases significantly with age. For example, approximately 26% of men under the age of 40 experience erectile dysfunction. Over the age of 75 it is already 77.5%.

Canguven O, Al Malki AH. **Vitamin D and Male Erectile Function: An Updated Review**. World J Mens Health. 2021;39(1):31-37. doi:10.5534/wjmh.190151

In this meta-analysis, the authors indicated a large role of vitamin D in male erectile function and that vitamin D deficiency is also associated with erectile dysfunction. They mentioned several important facts and mechanisms of vitamin D in this regard:
1. Vitamin D deficiency is associated with an increased erectile dysfunction (ED) prevalence. One study indicated that vitamin D levels below 20 ng/ml were associated with increased ED risk. In contrast, levels above 35 ng/ml were associated with decreased prevalence of ED.
2. Vitamin D is needed for the proper anatomical development of the penis during embryonal life.
3. Vitamin D regulates endothelial function and protects the endothelium from damage (e.g. caused by oxidative stress). Numerous studies have shown a link between vitamin D deficiency and endothelial dysfunction.
4. Vitamin D is able to stimulate nitric oxide (NO) production. NO is essential for vascular dilation, thus is also essential to penile erection.

5. As already mentioned, vitamin D plays a role in cardiovascular disease. These ailments are often related to ED. Hence, this vitamin is also important in erectile dysfunction.

6. Vitamin D is positively associated with total and bioavailable testosterone levels. Testosterone, in turn, modulates nearly every component involved in erectile function. Its deficiency is usually associated with ED.

7. ED is associated with inflammation. Vitamin D, as we already know, is known for its anti-inflammatory properties and in this case may protect the cells through suppressing inflammatory factors.

CHAPTER 31: CHRONIC RHINOSINUSITIS

Chronic rhinosinusitis is an inflammatory disease of the paranasal sinuses. This ailment affects 1% to 5% of the US population. Vitamin D, in turn, turns out to be beneficial also in this case, probably due to its anti-inflammatory properties. Studies have shown (one of them below) that vitamin D levels are significantly reduced in people with chronic rhinosinusitis and that supplementation helps to relieve unpleasant symptoms of this disease (nasal congestion, sneezing, nasal itching, and rhinorrhea).

Baruah, Binayak et al. **"The role of oral vitamin D3 supplementation in the treatment of Chronic Rhinosinusitis in adults with Vitamin D deficiency."** Journal of Family Medicine and Primary Care 9 (2020): 2877 - 2879.

Two hundred patients with chronic rhinosinusitis and vitamin D deficiency participated in the above study. One hundred people were given 60,000 IU (this comes to an average of about 8,500 IU per day) of vitamin D once a week for three months. At the beginning, the average level of vitamin D in these people was 12.31 ng/ml and increased after three months to 29.71 ng/ml. The second group of one hundred people was given a placebo. Scientists found that in the group supplementing vitamin D there was a significant reduction in the symptoms of chronic rhinosinusitis (as measured by the Total Nasal Symptom Score).

CHAPTER 32:
BONE HEALTH

The first thing people think of when they hear about vitamin D is bone health. This, indeed, is a correct thought. Vitamin D plays an extremely important role in musculoskeletal health. It promotes calcium absorption, mineralization of osteoid tissue formation in bone, and proper maintenance of muscle function. On the other hand, vitamin D deficiency leads to bone loss and muscle weakness. We will look at two studies that describe the effectiveness of this vitamin in more detail in these aspects.

Chapuy, Marie Claire et al. "**Vitamin D3 and calcium to prevent hip fractures in elderly women.**" The New England journal of medicine 327 23 (1992): 1637-42 .

The authors of this publication investigated the effect of vitamin D (800 IU/day) supplementation with calcium (tricalcium phosphate, containing 1.2 g of elemental calcium) on the frequency of hip fractures and other nonvertebral fractures in 3270 older women (mean age 84 years). The study lasted 18 months. In subjects who were treated with vitamin D and calcium, the number of hip fractures was 43% lower and the total number of nonvertebral fractures was 32% lower than among those who received placebo. Furthermore, the bone density of the proximal femur increased 2.7% in the vitamin D group whereas in the placebo group there was a 4.6% reduction.

Yao P, Bennett D, Mafham M, Lin X, Chen Z, Armitage J, Clarke R. **Vitamin D and Calcium for the Prevention of Fracture: A Systematic Review and Meta-analysis. JAMA Netw Open**. 2019 Dec 2;2(12):e1917789. doi: 10.1001/jamanetworkopen.2019.17789. PMID: 31860103; PMCID: PMC6991219.

In this systematic review and meta-analysis, scientists wanted to assess the risks of fractures associated with differences in vitamin D levels in observational studies as well as the same risk associated with vitamin D supplementation in randomized controlled trials. As it turned out, after analyzing 11 meta-analyzes with 39 141 participants, each increase of 10 ng/ml in 25(OH)D concentration was associated with a reduction of the risk for any fracture by 7% and for hip fracture by 20%. Additionally, a meta-analysis of 6 randomized controlled trials with 49,282 participants showed that vitamin D supplementation (yielding a median difference in 25(OH)D concentration of 9.2 ng/ml) along with calcium (daily doses of 1000-1200 mg) contributed to 6% risk reduction for any fracture and a 16% risk reduction for hip fracture.

CHAPTER 33: SLEEP

Good-quality sleep is the basis of health. Poor-quality sleep, on the other hand, can destroy health. A lack of good-quality sleep can lead to a variety of diseases. If this lack is chronic, the risk of very serious health consequences such as diabetes, obesity, depression, hypertension, heart attack, and stroke increases significantly. As studies have shown, vitamin D deficiency may be one of the causes of poor sleep quality. Therefore, also, if we feel that our sleep is not of the best quality, it may be worth checking the 25(OH)D levels and correcting them in the case of vitamin D deficiency.

Gao, Qi et al. **"The Association between Vitamin D Deficiency and Sleep Disorders: A Systematic Review and Meta-Analysis."** Nutrients 10 (2018): n. pag.

The authors of this meta-analysis of 9 studies (6 cross-sectional, 2 case-control, and 1 cohort studies) and 9,397 participants examined the relationship between vitamin D and sleep. By comparing the lowest levels with the highest levels of 25(OH)D in the subjects, they concluded that those with deficiencies had a significantly increased risk of sleep disorders. Additionally, vitamin D deficiency was associated with poor sleep quality, short sleep duration and sleepiness. According to the criteria suggested by the Institute of Medicine (IOM), when the vitamin D level was lower than 20 ng/ml, the risk of poor sleep quality increased by almost 60%.

CHAPTER 34: BPPV

Benign paroxysmal positional vertigo (BPPV) is a common inner ear disorder, which causes dizziness, unsteadiness and often nausea during the head position changes. Scientists have shown that vitamin D supplementation can reduce the number of recurrent attacks of benign paroxysmal positional vertigo.

Abdelmaksoud, Aida A. et al. **"Relation between vitamin D deficiency and benign paroxysmal positional vertigo."** Scientific Reports 11 (2021): n. pag.

Abdelmaksoud, et al, examined the effect of vitamin D deficiency on recurrent attacks in benign paroxysmal positional vertigo (BPPV). They enrolled 40 patients with this condition and with an average vitamin D level of 12.3 ng/ml. One group received 8000 IU of vitamin D daily for 2 weeks followed by 4000 IU daily for 2 weeks and then 8000 IU single dose weekly for 3 months in addition to canal repositioning maneuver, whereas the other group was treated with canal repositioning maneuver only. After 6 months, the level of vitamin D in the first group increased to 26.3 ng/ml, with no changes in the second group. It was found that the mean of recurrent attacks of BPPV in the first group was significantly lower than in the second group. The correlation between the recurrence rate of BPPV episodes and vitamin D was negative.

CHAPTER 35: HEADACHE AND MIGRAINE

Up to a billion people can suffer from migraines worldwide. More often this ailment (2-3 times) affects women than men. Sometimes the pain is so bad that we are unable to function normally. Then we usually reach for some painkillers as well. However, it turns out that the frequent use of pain medications for migraines can lead to even more frequent headaches. So we take headache medicine, feel relieved for a while, but then the headache comes back and intensifies. Therefore, it is important to look for the causes and eliminate them, not the symptoms. One of these causes of migraines may be vitamin D deficiency. There are many ways that can lead to this effect when we are deficient in vitamin D, ranging from excessive inflammation, sensitization of the second and third neurons, and low serum levels of magnesium.

Zhang, Yuan-feng et al. **"The Efficacy of Vitamin D Supplementation for Migraine: A Meta-Analysis of Randomized Controlled Studies."** Clinical Neuropharmacology (2021): n. pag.

The above publications from 2021 indicated that people who supplemented with vitamin D had significantly fewer headache attacks, headache days per month and reduced headache severity. The Migraine Disability Assessment (MIDAS), which helps to assess the extent to which migraines affect functioning in normal life, was also lower. Researchers concluded their research that vitamin D is effective to alleviate migraine.

Liampas, Ioannis et al. **"Vitamin D serum levels in patients with migraine: A meta-analysis."** Revue neurologique (2020): n. pag.

Liampas, et al, in their meta-analysis of eight studies concluded: "25(OH)D concentration is lower in patients with migraine than healthy individuals. In view of this finding, investigation of the effect of vitamin D supplementation in patients suffering from migraine is warranted."

Peikert, Andreas et al. **"Prophylaxis of Migraine with Oral Magnesium: Results From A Prospective, Multi-Center, Placebo-Controlled and Double-Blind Randomized Study."** Cephalalgia 16 (1996): 257 - 263.

Low vitamin D levels can reduce the absorption of magnesium in the gut. This mineral, on the other hand, has been shown to be very effective in treating headaches and migraines. For example, in the above study, 81 patients aged 18-65 years were included. People were given 600 mg of magnesium (trimagnesium dicitrate) or a placebo daily for 12 weeks. In weeks 9-12 the attack frequency was reduced by 41.6% in the magnesium group. The number of days with migraine and the drug consumption for symptomatic treatment decreased significantly. Duration and intensity of the attacks also decreased compared to placebo.

CHAPTER 36:
DEPRESSION

Vitamin D can help treat depression. According to WHO approximately 300 million people in the world suffer from this disease. Various other sources give even higher numbers. In addition, nearly 800,000 people die by suicide each year. Vitamin D can reduce this statistic for several reasons. Vitamin D is involved in various biochemical processes and has an effect on such hormones as serotonin, dopamine and noradrenaline. Serotonin, for example, regulates mood, behavior, and sleep. High levels of this hormone help us relax. In depression, serotonin levels are low. Vitamin D, in turn, plays a crucial role in the synthesis of this hormone. Dopamine is a so-called chemical of pleasure. Vitamin D promotes the gene expression of tyrosine hydroxylase. This enzyme, influences the synthesis of dopamine and norepinephrine (noradrenaline). With the second neurotransmitter, its low levels can lead to depression. Moreover, receptors for vitamin D are also present on neurons and glia in brain areas such as the cingulate cortex and hippocampus. These areas have been linked to depression. Overall, vitamin D is also involved in brain development, neuroprotection, neuroplasticity and neuroimmunomodulation of the brain.

Anglin, Rebecca E. S. et al. **"Vitamin D deficiency and depression in adults: systematic review and meta-analysis."** British Journal of Psychiatry 202 (2013): 100 - 107.

A meta-analysis of 31,424 participants showed that people with depression had lower vitamin D levels than the control group. Those with lower levels of this vitamin had an increased risk of depression by up to 31%.

Spedding, S. (2014). **Vitamin D and Depression: A Systematic**

Review and Meta-Analysis Comparing Studies with and without Biological Flaws. Nutrients, 6, 1501 - 1518.

Another scientific publication indicated that vitamin D supplementation helps with depression. The authors also found that the results of using vitamin D may be comparable to the use of antidepressants. Vitamin D doses in the various analyzed studies varied from 400 IU to 18,400 IU.

Khoraminya, Nayereh et al. **"Therapeutic effects of vitamin D as adjunctive therapy to fluoxetine in patients with major depressive disorder."** Australian & New Zealand Journal of Psychiatry 47 (2013): 271 - 275.

Vitamin D also turned out to be effective along with other antidepressants. In this double-blind, randomized, placebo-controlled trial, one group took 1500 IU of vitamin D plus 20 mg of fluoxetine and the other group took only fluoxetine. The study lasted 8 weeks. After this time, it was found that the results of controlling depressive symptoms when using vitamin D with fluoxetine were significantly better than using fluoxetine alone.

Mozaffari-khosravi, Hassan et al. **"The Effect of 2 Different Single Injections of High Dose of Vitamin D on Improving the Depression in Depressed Patients With Vitamin D Deficiency: A Randomized Clinical Trial."** Journal of Clinical Psychopharmacology 33 (2013): 378–385.

In the above study scientists examined the effect of single injections of high dose of vitamin D on improving depression in depressed patients with vitamin D deficiency. Participants were randomly assigned to 3 groups of 40. One group got an intramuscular single dose of 300,000 IU of vitamin D, the second group got 150,000 IU, and the third group got nothing. After three months, various parameters were measured. There was a significant difference in mean of Beck Depression Inventory II test score between the first group and third one (It is a very popular psychometric test for measuring the severity of depression). That is, the correction of vitamin D deficiency improved depression. Additionally, it was found that a single dose of 300,000 IU of vitamin D had been more effective than 150,000 IU.

CHAPTER 37:
FATIGUE

Fatigue is a common symptom in our world today. It can lead to a significant decrease in the quality of life, a decrease in well-being and productivity. Doctors often prescribe various supplements to this complaint, including iron or vitamin D. As I am about to show, prescribing vitamin D is not unfounded in this case.

Johnson, K., & Sattari, M. (2015). **Vitamin D deficiency and fatigue: an unusual presentation**. SpringerPlus, 4.

This publication presents a case of a 61 year old man suffering from excessive daytime fatigue. None of the features he reported indicated depression or anxiety. He also detailed good sleep hygiene and 7-8 hours a day sleeping (without sleep apnea). A comprehensive examination, including testosterone levels or thyroid function, showed no abnormalities. However, serum 25(OH)D level was very low, at 18.4 ng/ml. For this reason, it was decided to increase the patient's vitamin D level. Vitamin D supplementation was initiated with 50000 IU of ergocholecalciferol (vitamin D2) weekly for 8 weeks, followed by 1000 IU of vitamin D daily. Improvement of fatigue and daytime appeared after 2 weeks. Moreover, complete resolution of his symptoms was achieved within 3 months.

Of course, this is not the only example of vitamin D's effects on fatigue. I have heard about such activity of vitamin D many times from doctors I know. I know this from my own body experiences as well. What's more, there are also publications like the one below.

Nowak, Albina et al. "**Effect of vitamin D3 on self-perceived fatigue**." Medicine 95 (2016): n. pag.

In this double-blind placebo-controlled clinical trial, scientists investigated the effect of vitamin D on 120 otherwise healthy people with fatigue and low vitamin D levels (below 20 ng/ml). One group received 100,000 IU of a single oral dose of vitamin D, while the other group received a placebo. After four weeks, in the vitamin D supplementation group, the mean FAS (The Fatigue Assessment Scale) decreased significantly more than in the placebo group. A similar trend emerged with amelioration of fatigue. Overall, the improvement in fatigue was associated with an increase in 25(OH)D levels.

CHAPTER 38:
MICROBIOME

Health is said to start in the gut. There is a lot of truth in this. Although we still know little and are just starting to explore the gut, we already know that a healthy gut is the basis of health. More and more often we also hear what is good and bad for our intestines and our microbiota, what to eat and what to avoid. And rightly so. However, one factor is rarely mentioned which may also play a crucial role in gut health. Vitamin D is this factor. The following 2020 study showed just such activity of vitamin D.

Charoenngam, Nipith et al. **"The Effect of Various Doses of Oral Vitamin D3 Supplementation on Gut Microbiota in Healthy Adults: A Randomized, Double-blinded, Dose-response Study."** AntiCancer Research 40 (2019): 551 - 556.

The purpose of this randomized, double-blinded, dose-response study was to examine the effect of vitamin D supplementation on gut microbiota. Twenty adults with vitamin D levels below 30 ng/ml were enrolled in the study. They got respectively; 600, 4,000 or 10,000 IU per day of oral vitamin D. To identify the gut microbiota, stool samples were collected at baseline and also at week 8. Increased relative abundance of Akkermansia (Akkermansia municiphila, for example, has been shown to be associated with decreased risk of cancer, obesity and atherosclerosis) was associated with higher serum 25(OH)D levels. Moreover a significant decrease in Firmicutes to Bacteroidetes (F/B) ratio was observed (high F/B ratio, among others, has been linked to obesity). Researchers also observed a dose-dependent increase in the relative abundance of Bacteroides and Parabacteroides (both of these bacteria are associated with alleviating intestinal inflammation by helping to maintain the expansion of regulatory T cells). In the words of the authors themselves: "In conclusion, we observed that an increase in baseline serum 25(OH)D levels was correlated with increased bacteria associated with decreased risk of cardiovascular and metabolic diseases, obesity, and cancers. We also found that increased baseline 25(OH)D levels were inversely correlated with decreased periodondopathic bacteria. After 8 weeks of vitamin D supplementation, we observed an alteration of gut microbiota towards a decrease in Firmicutes to Bacteroidetes ratio, which is an indicator associated with obesity and metabolic syndrome. Finally, we observed a dose-dependent increase in bacteria associated with decreased inflammatory bowel disease activity in response to various doses of vitamin D3 supplementation." and even shorter "increased serum 25(OH)D was associated with increased beneficial bacteria and decreased pathogenic bacteria."

CHAPTER 39: LIFESPAN

Vitamin D affects our lifespan. Since I mentioned the remarkable effects of vitamin D in maintaining and restoring health, this information may seem obvious. However, here I would like to add something a little different that takes place on a different level and is unknown to most people.

But first, a little explanation. There are telomeres at both ends of each chromosome. These are specific DNA-protein structures, which, for example, protect the genome from nucleolytic degradation or unnecessary recombination. With age, the length of the telomeres becomes shorter. The telomere length can therefore serve as some measure of our lifespan. Telomerase, on the other hand, is an enzyme that helps maintain telomere length. And here our vitamin matters.

Zhu, H. et al. "**Increased telomerase activity and vitamin D supplementation in overweight African Americans.**" International Journal of Obesity 36 (2012): 805-809.

In this study, people were given 60,000 IU per month (equal to about 2,000 IU per day) of oral vitamin D supplementation. In the vitamin D group, PBMC telomerase activity increased by 19.2% from baseline. The change in activity was significant. In the placebo group, the PBMC telomerase activity did not change. The results therefore showed that vitamin D may also have a life-extending effect on the DNA level, which is associated with increased activation of telomerase.

CHAPTER 40:
PREGNANCY

As most of us have or will have children, the information in this section cannot be overestimated. I will show in a moment that vitamin D is absolutely essential to prevent many complications of pregnancy such as preeclampsia, gestational diabetes, cesarean section, craniotabes, and preterm labor. Furthermore, we will see that if the mother is getting enough vitamin D, there is no need to supplement the infant. Let's begin.

Hollis, Bruce W et al. "**Vitamin D supplementation during pregnancy: Double-blind, randomized clinical trial of safety and effectiveness.**" Journal of Bone and Mineral Research 26 (2011): n. pag.

In this double-blind, randomized clinical trial from 2002 women with a singleton pregnancy at 12–16 weeks' gestation received 400, 2000 or 4000 IU vitamin D per day until delivery (depending on initial level of 25(OH)D). Women with levels below 40 ng/ml got 400 IU, 2000 IU or 4000 IU, those with levels between 40-60 ng/ml 400IU or 2000 IU, and those with levels above 60 ng/ml 400 IU. The primary goal of this study was to test safety and effectiveness through vitamin D supplementation. 4,000 IU per day proved to be safe and the most effective in achieving sufficiency in all women and their neonates. However, as it turned out, vitamin D had an significant effect on some birth outcomes (such vitamin D activities were not known 20 years ago yet). Due to vitamin D, there was a reduction in the number of cesarean sections, preeclampsia, gestational diabetes as well as comorbidities of pregnancy.

Craniotabes is a disease associated with severe vitamin D deficiency. It is a significant softening or demineralized area of the skull in infants. As it has been shown, many of these children have severe vitamin D deficiencies, even below 10 ng/ml. Fortunately, it's a condition that can be normalized with this vitamin and calcium supplementation.

Wagner, Carol L. et al. "**Vitamin D administration during pregnancy as prevention for pregnancy, neonatal and postnatal complications.**" Reviews in Endocrine and Metabolic Disorders 18 (2017): 307-322.

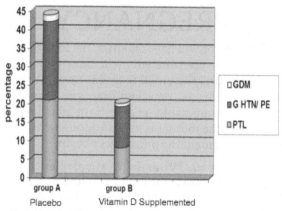

Adapted from: SablokA, et al. Clinical Endocrinology 2015; 83: 536.

"Effect of vitamin D supplementation starting at 20 weeks of pregnancy with respect to the development of complications of pregnancy. Pregnancy complication in the form of preterm labor (PTL), gestational hypertension (GHTN)/preeclampsia (PE) or gestational diabetes mellitus (GDM) were observed in 25/57 (44%) women taking placebo compared to 22/108 (20.4%) women being supplemented with vitamin D. Significance between groups was p < 0.02."

As shown above, vitamin D supplementation starting at 20 weeks of pregnancy was associated with a much smaller incidence of complications of pregnancy.

Moreover, analysis of several results showed that gestational age at birth does not normalize until 40-50 ng/ml. In other words, vitamin D has a strong effect in preventing preterm births. The risk reduction can be as high as 59% comparing levels above 40 ng/ml to levels below 20 ng/ml.

Other studies have noted that preeclampsia (characterized by high blood pressure and protein in their urine) hardly occurs at all in women who have levels above 40 ng/ml during pregnancy. In addition, there seems also to be a link between vitamin D and the pain of labor. As vitamin D levels increase, the intensity of labor pain decreases drastically. Again, levels of at least 40-50 ng/ml are desirable for this to happen. In my previous book, I also mentioned a study involving 400 women. Women with adequate vitamin D levels had a four-fold lower risk of having surgery in childbirth.

Wagner, Carol L. et al. **"High-dose vitamin D3 supplementation in a cohort of breastfeeding mothers and their infants: a 6-month follow-up pilot study**." Breastfeeding medicine : the official journal of the Academy of Breastfeeding Medicine 1 2 (2006): 59-70 .

Lactating women at one month postpartum were enrolled in this randomized-control pilot trial. They were divided into two groups. In the first group, women got 400 IU/day and their infants got 300 IU. In the second, they got 6400 IU and infants receive a placebo. Vitamin D was administered for 6 months. As the study found, the vitamin D status of an infant supplementing oral vitamin D at a dose of 300 IU/day was comparable to that of a child who only received vitamin D from the mother who supplemented the 6,400 IU dose. In women supplementing with 400 IU of vitamin D and having a level of about 35 ng/ml, only about 70 IU/l was passed into the milk. On the other hand, a child who drank milk from a mother who had a 25(OH)D level above 50 ng/ml as a result of regular supplementation of 6400 IU/day, could receive 400-600 IU of vitamin D with this milk.

Here we can conclude that if the mother takes care of the right amount of vitamin D, there is no need to give the infant this vitamin in the form of a supplement. The baby will simply get it through the mother's milk. It is worth mentioning that of the amount consumed by the mother, the child will get about 8-10%. For example, when the mother consumes 8,000 IU of vitamin D, the child will get 640-800 IU of this vitamin. In nursing women, the doctors say, this dose should be at least 6,000 IU so that supplementation is not needed. It should also always be remembered that doses up to 10,000 IU per day and levels up to 100 ng/ml in this case (as in any other) are simply normal in human physiology. There is no need to worry. But more on that later.

CHAPTER 41: OTHER RELEVANT SUBSTANCES

However, it's not just the dose that affects whether this vitamin is effective or not. Vitamin D also needs many other nutrients to work properly. These substances will help the body to create an active form of vitamin D. Only this form has a pro-health effect on our organism. Furthermore, some substances contribute to the fact that once we have a high level of this vitamin, we will not experience any side effects. This is what this chapter will be about; both about the substances necessary for the body to produce an active form of vitamin D and about substances that enable safe supplementation.

Magnesium

Tanaka, Kiyoshi et al. **"Insufficiency of B vitamins with its possible clinical implications."** Journal of Clinical Biochemistry and Nutrition 67 (2020): 19 - 25.

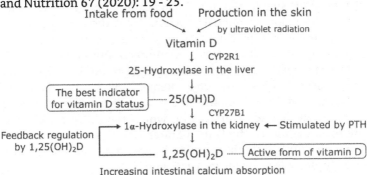

Uwitonze, A.M., & Razzaque, M.S. (2018). **Role of Magnesium in Vitamin D Activation and Function. Journal of Osteopathic Medicine Journal of Osteopathic Medicine,** 118, 181 - 189.

As we can see in the picture above, vitamin D metabolism is not the simplest. First, 7-dehydrocholesterol on our skin, under the influence of UVB, will be converted into vitamin D (cholecalciferol). We can also receive this vitamin D (in the form of cholecalciferol) in a supplement or from food. There is not much difference here (as can be seen at the top of the picture). Then vitamin D (cholecalciferol) is converted in the liver to 25(OH)D. It is by measuring the level of 25(OH)D that we can best assess the status of vitamin D in the body. The last step will be the transformation of 25(OH)D in the kidney into the active form of vitamin D, i.e. 1.25(OH)2D. So we already have our vitamin in its powerful form. But, someone may ask what is the relationship of magnesium with this. The shortest answer - huge. All the enzymes that metabolize vitamin D seem to require magnesium. This element acts as a cofactor in the enzymatic reactions both in the liver and kidneys. However, that's not all we know about magnesium in the case of vitamin D. As proven magnesium supplementation reduces the resistance to vitamin D treatment and interestingly, some studies show that this element may determine the number of vitamin D receptors. Another aspect of magnesium is, in turn, its protective effect against excess calcium. As we know, vitamin D increases the intestinal calcium absorption. And it is mainly this excess of calcium that is the fear of vitamin D supplementation. Magnesium, on the other hand, is a calcium blocker, removes calcium from the bloodstream as well as removes intracellular calcium. Hence, with higher doses of vitamin D, supplementation with magnesium may also turn out to be crucial. At preventive dosages (or rather levels), dietary magnesium is likely to suffice. Remember, the standard diet in the United States contains about 50% of the Recommended Daily Allowance for magnesium, which ranges from 320-420 mg for an adult. In the United States, about 68% are deficient in magnesium. Essentially, in food, the amount of magnesium already decreased between 1940 and 1991, by 15% to 26%, depending on the product. Moreover, due to heavy chemical fertilization and the effects of the Green Revolution, the current situation looks even worse. Therefore, it should be remembered that this diet really should contain foods rich in magnesium.

Vitamin K2

Vitamin K2 is a substance that is not necessary for vitamin D supplementation, but at high doses may show a protective effect. Vitamin K2 increases the production of Matrix Gla Protein (MGP), which regulates calcium in the body. Vitamin K2 can prevent calcium accumulation in soft tissues as well as blood vessels, which is where calcium should not be. On the other hand, if we lack vitamin K2, calcium does not end up in the bones or teeth and begins to build up on the walls of the arteries. Studies have already shown that people who supplement with vitamin K2 have an over 50% lower risk of severe aortic calcification and an over 40% lower risk of coronary heart disease. In addition, supplementation with vitamin K2 turns out to be very effective in the prevention and treatment of fractures, osteoporosis and osteomalacia. All this is related to the calcium-regulating effect of vitamin K2. Therefore, vitamin K2 supplementation is reasonable when taking high doses of vitamin D, which consequently result in higher calcium absorption and higher calcium levels. It is considered that 100 mcg of vitamin K2-MK7 per 10,000 IU of vitamin D is optimal.

Zinc

Another essential nutrient is zinc. Zinc is a part of over 600 enzymes over 2500 transcription factors and numerous proteins. Also, in the functioning of vitamin D, this element plays an important role.

Amos, A., & Razzaque, M.S. (2022). **Zinc and its role in vitamin D function.** Current Research in Physiology, 5, 203 - 207.

"Zinc modulates the structure and binding of the DNA binding domain of the 1,25-dihydroxycholecalciferol response element DNA; therefore, without zinc, proper VDR (Vitamin D Receptor) structural conformation cannot be formed. Therefore, the activity of vitamin D-dependent genes relies on zinc, making zinc an essential cofactor for vitamin D activity."

Zinc is an important cofactor for vitamin D and its deficiency has a negative effect on vitamin D receptor expression. The conclusion of this study would therefore explain why some other studies have established that zinc deficiency was the strongest predictor of vitamin D deficiency in a studied population.

Boron

Studies have shown that boron, among others, is able to extend the half-life of vitamin D. For this reason, it is worth ensuring that this valuable element is not missing in the diet. Boron can be found in significant amounts, for example, in almonds, peanut butter, walnuts and Brazil nuts, beans, broccoli and carrots.

Note: vitamin A & E

Maurya, V.K., & Aggarwal, M. (2017). **Factors influencing the absorption of vitamin D in GIT: an overview. Journal of Food Science and Technology,** 54, 3753-3765.

When taking high doses of fat-soluble vitamins at once, one vitamin may reduce the absorption of the other due to a similar absorption mechanism. For example, high concentration of vitamin A may reduce bioavailability of vitamin D by 30%. A similar relationship applies to vitamin E. Vitamin E can impair the vitamin D absorption from 15% at medium concentration to 17% at high concentration. Nonetheless, I would like to emphasize at this point that the above facts should not be a cause for concern when it comes to normal supplementation or regular meals. If for some reason we take large amounts of vitamins A, D, E, it is worth taking them separately.

CHAPTER 42: WHAT ELSE TO REMEMBER

Being overweight is a big obstacle for vitamin D to function properly. As we already know, vitamin D is a fat-soluble vitamin. Obese people naturally have more fat. One of the most important reasons obese people have lower vitamin D levels is that their adipose tissue absorbs this fat-soluble vitamin. Vitamin D just needs to be in the blood to be effective. This applies to both vitamin D from supplements and that produced after exposure to sunlight. Hence, It is therefore understood that researchers have shown that one excessive BMI unit induces a 1.15% reduction in the 25(OH)D concentration. It can be seen in the statistics.

Zakharova, Irina N. et al. **"Vitamin D Insufficiency in Overweight and Obese Children and Adolescents."** Frontiers in Endocrinology 10 (2019): n. pag.

Vitamin D levels are below 30 ng/ml in a significant number of overweight children and adults: 78% in the United States, 96% in Germany and 92% in Russia. Overall, in obese people, the prevalence of vitamin D deficiency is approximately 35 percent higher than in non-obese people.

Holick, Michael F et al. **"Evaluation, treatment, and prevention of vitamin D deficiency: an Endocrine Society clinical practice guideline**." The Journal of clinical endocrinology and metabolism 96 7 (2011): 1911-30 .

When obese and nonobese adults were exposed to simulated sunlight or received an oral dose of vitamin D, blood levels of vitamin D in obese adults went up by no more than 50% compared with nonobese adults. Thus, these results indicated that obese people require significantly higher doses of vitamin D to achieve the same vitamin D levels as non-obese people.

Older people are also more likely to develop vitamin D deficiency.

Gallagher, J.C. (2013). **Vitamin D and aging. Endocrinology and metabolism clinics of North America**, 42 2, 319-32 .

"There is a decrease in the concentration of 7-dehydrocholesterol in the epidermis in old compared with young individuals and a reduced response to UV light, resulting in a 50% decrease in the formation of previtamin D3."
Moreover, the reduction in the production of 1,25(OH)2D on a similar scale is also due to an age-related decline in renal function. For these reasons, the dose for the elderly should be at least twice as high. However, in the event of obesity and the age of over 75 years, the dose should be even 4 times higher.

What seems also important and rarely mentioned, high consumption of fructose can decrease serum levels of 1,25(OH)2D (the active form of the vitamin). This effect has been observed in both rodents and humans and is related to the influence of fructose on the metabolism of vitamin D. For this reason, people who eat a lot of sweets or drink a lot of fruit juices should be careful as it may affect their vitamin D levels.

NOTE: There is also a certain significant difference between vitamin D3 and D2 to be aware of as well. When I write vitamin D in a book, it refers to vitamin D3, not vitamin D2. Vitamin D(3) or cholecalciferol is largely used in studies and this form is also found mainly in supplements. If vitamin D2 was used in some study, I emphasized it.

Heaney, Robert Proulx et al. **"Vitamin D(3) is more potent than vitamin D(2) in humans."** The Journal of clinical endocrinology and metabolism 96 3 (2011): E447-52 .

It turns out that vitamin D3 is 87% more potent in raising 25(OH)D than vitamin D2. Furthermore, vitamin D3 contributes to a 2-3 times greater storage of this vitamin. Consequently, if we take vitamin D2 we must take much higher doses to achieve the same 25(OH)D level as would be required by taking vitamin D(3).

CHAPTER 43: SAFETY OF VITAMIN D

It is impossible to determine one level of vitamin D, after which all people will experience the toxic effects of vitamin D supplementation. This is mainly due to the fact that everyone is slightly different and their body functions differently. We can only analyze scientific publications and try to outline some trends and directions; what levels can be safe and what already pose a certain risk. We will try to do this.

Jones, Glenville. "**Pharmacokinetics of vitamin D toxicity.**" The American journal of clinical nutrition 88 2 (2008): 582S-586S .

"Although current data support the viewpoint that the biomarker plasma 25(OH)D concentration must rise above 750 nmol/L (300 ng/ml) to produce vitamin D toxicity, the more prudent upper limit of 250 nmol/L might be retained to ensure a wide safety margin."
Studies suggest that vitamin D concentrations in serum lower than 300 ng/ml do not induce any toxicity.

Kimball, Samantha M. et al. "**Evaluation of vitamin D3 intakes up to 15,000 international units/day and serum 25-hydroxyvitamin D concentrations up to 300 nmol/L on calcium metabolism in a community setting.**" Dermato-endocrinology 9 (2017): n. pag.

"While the present study does not address what is an optimal vitamin D status, it does confirm the safety of serum 25(OH)D concentrations up to 300 nmol/L (120 ng/ml) and intakes of vitamin D up to 15,000 IU/d. Further, the results presented here demonstrate a variable response to vitamin D intake and suggest that intakes of 6,000–8,000 IU/d are required to achieve serum 25(OH)D above 100 nmol/L (40 ng/ml)."

This study showed that vitamin D levels below 120 ng/ml as well as a daily vitamin D intake of up to 15,000 IU per day were not associated with any toxicity. The authors found that at least 6000-8000 IU is required to exceed the 40 ng/ml level. However, approximately 10,000 IU vitamin D per day is required to achieve a more desirable level such as, for example, 60 ng/ml.

McCullough, P.J., & Amend, J. (2017). **Results of daily oral dosing with up to 60,000 international units (iu) of vitamin D3 for 2 to 6 years in 3 adult males.** The Journal of Steroid Biochemistry and Molecular Biology, 173, 308-312.

A 2011 report showed that hypercalcemia resolved when the 25(OH)D levels of two patients dropped below 400 ng/ml after these individuals accidentally hit levels from 645 ng/ml to 1220 ng/ml. In the above report, another three cases were noted. In the first case, for 6 years (from April 2009), a person took increasingly higher doses of vitamin D from 6,500 IU/day to 60,000 IU/day (including 20,000 IU for 24 months; 40,000 IU for 12 months; 50,000 IU for 10 months, and 60,000 IU since October 2014). This person's vitamin D levels were 28, 81, 204, 216, 225, 166, and 218ng/ml. In the second case, the person took from 10,000 IU to 30,000 IU for almost 4 years. This person's 25(OH)D levels were 96.6, 161.1 and 106.9ng/ml. Additionally, this subject reported marked clinical improvement in asthma. In the third case, the person supplemented from 10,000 IU to 20,000 IU of vitamin D per day. This person's vitamin D levels were 31.4, 102, 164, 148, and 143ng/ml. Importantly, no one developed hypercalcemia or any adverse events.

CHAPTER 44:
OPTIMAL VITAMIN
D LEVELS

Haddad, J.G., & Chyu, K.J. (1971). **Competitive protein-binding radioassay for 25-hydroxycholecalciferol**. The Journal of clinical endocrinology and metabolism, 33 6, 992-5 .

Group	No.	Age	Consumption of D weekly (units)	Weekly exposure to sunlight (hours)	Plasma 25(OH)D (ng/ml)
Normal Volunteers	40	30.2	2230	8.8	27.3
Biliary Cirrhosis	4	1.5 - 55	2500	_____	6.4
Lifeguards	8	18.5	2895	53	64.4

Back in 1971 authors of this publication measured vitamin D levels in normal volunteers, people with biliary cirrhosis, and lifeguards. They chose people with biliary cirrhosis because it is a condition characterized by fat malabsorption, which should affect the absorption of fat-soluble vitamin D. Normal volunteers were office workers, doctors, teachers etc. In those people who were not significantly exposed to sunlight, the mean vitamin D level was only 27.3 ng/ml. On the other hand, there were lifeguards who were exposed to sunlight, just like we humans in our evolution. In this case, the body could produce as much vitamin D as it needed until the level was over 60 ng/ml. Unfortunately, often, more than 50 years later, we look at those 30 ng/ml and think these are the right levels. The recommended dose of vitamin D is 2000 IU or sometimes even less. Interestingly, on the other hand, a person after sun exposure can produce up to 10 times as much, i.e. 20,000 IU/day.

How to do this? How to properly use the wonderful sun? It is not enough just to go outside. There are a few important things to know. As I wrote at the very beginning, only UVB light allows us to produce vitamin D. At that time, the angle of the sun has to be greater than 45°. Hence, here in Paris, the possibility of natural synthesis of vitamin D from the sun occurs from around April to September. It is different in the United States and different in Great Britain. The highest angle of the sun, i.e. the most appropriate, is between 11 a.m and 1 p.m. Naturally, the closer we get to the equator, the more part of the year and more hours of the day we will be able to produce vitamin D. In turn, at latitudes of 45 ° or higher (Norway, Sweden, Canada etc.) the possibility of producing vitamin D is very limited. Though we already know when to go out into the sun, we still need to know how. The more body we have uncovered, the better, we can be in a swimsuit, for example. It is also not about long sunbathing, but e.g. for 15 minutes we expose the front of the body and 15 minutes the back of the body. No more is needed. Needless to say, it should be done regularly. If this is not possible (as in most cases), vitamin D supplementation should most likely be considered. The doses do not matter, what matters is the 25(OH)D level. Everyone can aim for a different level of vitamin D, especially in the case of illness. Moreover, for everyone, the same dose can raise vitamin D levels at different rates. This is important. In the previous chapter, I wrote a little about how much it should be approximately taken to achieve a particular level of vitamin D. The key word here is "approximately". I encourage everyone to measure the level of 25(OH)D both before and after supplementation. This will help determine what dose is necessary for us on a daily basis to maintain the appropriate level, a level that will largely protect us against various diseases and that will have a therapeutic effect when we already have some disease. But how high is this level supposed to be?

Based on the scientific studies I mentioned in this book and knowledge of human nature, we can conclude that the optimal (i.e. preventive) level of vitamin D is from about 60 ng/ml to 100 ng/ml. It is primarily a physiological level, i.e. achievable through sun exposure. Moreover, it is a vitamin D level that can reduce the risk of virtually all of the diseases discussed in this book. Very often this level will also contribute to the improvement of symptoms once the disease is there, and sometimes even to the complete disappearance of the disease. Nevertheless, for some diseases, levels of 100 ng/ml to 150 ng/ml and possibly more may be required to obtain the desired results. There were already examples in the book that indicated this. After the earlier chapter on the safety of vitamin D and the entire book, we can conclude that vitamin D is a rather very safe substance and therapy with higher doses of vitamin D will also be safe (especially when accompanied by other substances; at least vitamin K2 and magnesium). However, certainly, after exceeding 200 ng/ml or 300 ng/ml, it is worth testing the levels of calcium in the blood.

PART II: VITAMIN C

CHAPTER 45:
CANCER

As with vitamin D, the first disease we will deal with will be cancer, because it also causes the greatest fear in humans. The number of different therapies is endless; some are more effective and some are less effective, others are not effective at all. The topic of vitamin C treatment for cancer is at least controversial. Many people, when they hear about the treatment of cancer with vitamin C, do not believe it and often just laugh at the person who says such things. Many, if not most, doctors also unfortunately belong to this group. However, is it a matter of faith? And how many of them have even made the effort to study it? Because, especially in the last few years, there have been many new publications on this subject, and there will be even more, due to the results obtained. These results turn out to be very promising, which I will try to present in this chapter. What's more, we already know quite a lot why this is so. We already know some mechanisms of action. There are many of them by which vitamin C may prove beneficial in the prevention as well as treatment of cancer. We will start by briefly describing these mechanisms.

1. Vitamin C shows pro-oxidative activity in cancer cells, which induces cytotoxicity associated with hydrogen peroxide. Importantly, this activity does not adversely affect normal cells. Vitamin C promotes reduction of iron from Fe^{3+} to Fe^{2+} in the body. Fe^{2+}, in turn, reacts with H_2O_2 (Fenton reaction) to form the damaging hydroxyl radical (OH ·). The resulting oxidative stress can destroy cancer cells. Accordingly, high doses of vitamin C lead to DNA, protein and lipid damage of cancer cells (by increasing ROS). Studies has shown that the concentration of vitamin C must, however, be high (0.5-20 mM).

2. Vitamin C is essential in the process of collagen formation. Increased levels of this main component of connective tissue

can result in a reduction of metastasis. Such action has already been confirmed by preclinical studies and case report studies. Additionally, vitamin C also inhibits epithelial-mesenchymal-transition (EMT), which is involved in tumor progression and contributes to metastasis.

3. Vitamin C regulates the function of HIF hydroxylases, which deactivate HIF-1. Many studies have shown strong correlation between high levels of HIF-1 and tumor metastasis, poor patient prognosis and angiogenesis (the growth of tumor new blood vessels). Higher levels of tumor vitamin C were found to be inversely correlated with HIF-1 pathway activation.

4. Vitamin C induces TET dependent DNA demethylation. DNA methylation (reverse reaction to demethylation) is a crucial factor in the development of cancer and its aberrant patterns are common in this disease. Vitamin C, in turn, is essential for optimal TET enzyme activity. This activity has been recognized as a significant tumor suppressor mechanism in cancer.

Miller, P.G., & Ebert, B.L. (2017). **Leukaemia: Vitamin C regulates stem cells and cancer.** Nature, 549, 462-464.

For example, in acute myeloid leukemia TET2 mutations are common. Therefore, it can be assumed that vitamin C deficiency will accelerate leukemia because of the impairment of TET2 function.

Of course, these are not all the potential mechanisms of vitamin C in cancer, but they are some of the most important. Now let's dive into the studies showing the promising effect of vitamin C in this disease. We'll start with observational studies, two studies starting the era of vitamin C in cancer, and animal studies.

Observational studies

Michels, K.B., L. Holmberg, L. Bergkvist, et al. **"Dietary Antioxidant Vitamins, Retinol, and Breast Cancer Incidence in a Cohort of Swedish Women."** Intl J Cancer 91:4 (2001): 563–567.

To see if antioxidant vitamins can protect against breast cancer, researchers analyzed a large population-based prospective cohort study of Sweden that comprised 59.036 aged 40-76 years women. The women were free of cancer at baseline. During follow-up, 1,271 cases of invasive breast cancer were diagnosed.

As it turned out, women who were overweight and with the highest vitamin C consumption were found to have a 39% lower risk of breast cancer compared to women with the lowest consumption.

Zhang, S., D.J. Hunter, M.R. Forman, et al. **"Dietary Carotenoids and Vitamins A, C, and E and Risk of Breast Cancer."** J Natl Cancer Inst 91:6 (1999): 547–556.

This study examined the relationship between intakes of specific carotenoids, vitamins A, C, and E, consumption of fruits and vegetables, and risk of breast cancer. The observation included 83234 women aged 33-60 years in 1980. Through 1994, they identified 2697 invasive breast cancer cases (784 premenopausal and 1913 postmenopausal). Premenopausal women who consumed an average of 205 mg of vitamin C per day had a 63% reduced risk of breast cancer compared with those women with an average intake of 70 mg.

Harris, Holly R. et al. **"Vitamin C intake and breast cancer mortality in a cohort of Swedish women."** British Journal of Cancer 109 (2013): 257 - 264.

A similar relationship between vitamin C and breast cancer has been observed in a cohort of Swedish women. Here, the study included 3,405 women diagnosed with invasive breast cancer. From 1987-2010, there were 1055 total deaths with 416 deaths from breast cancer. Women whose pre-diagnosis vitamin C intake was the highest had a 25% lower risk of breast cancer death than women who consumed the least vitamin C. Moreover, it seemed that such a relationship also applied to total mortality and accounted for 16%.

Fan, Hua et al. **"Association between vitamin C intake and the risk of pancreatic cancer: a meta-analysis of observational studies**." Scientific Reports 5 (2015): n. pag.

The authors of this meta-analysis aimed to investigate the association between the intake of vitamin C and risk of pancreatic cancer. For this purpose, they analyzed the data from 17 studies including 4827 pancreatic cancer cases. Scientists additionally made a distinction between populations including; Caucasian, Asian and Mixed. The analysis showed that the highest vitamin C intakes are significantly associated with reduced risk of pancreatic cancer compared to the lowest vitamin C intakes. This risk can be reduced by approximately 30% to 42%.

Luo, Jie et al. **"Association between vitamin C intake and lung cancer: a dose-response meta-analysis."** Scientific Reports 4 (2014): n. pag.

The authors of this publication investigated the association between the intake of vitamin C and lung cancer risk. They analyzed eighteen articles reporting 21 studies involving 8938 lung cancer cases. They found a significant link between vitamin C levels and the risk of lung cancer. Additionally, this link was linear and dose-response. As it turned out, for every 100-milligram increase in daily vitamin C intake among men, the risk of developing lung cancer decreased by 7%.

Pioneering publications

Cameron, E., & Pauling, L.C. (1978). **Supplemental ascorbate in the supportive treatment of cancer: reevaluation of prolongation of survival times in terminal human cancer.** Proceedings of the National Academy of Sciences of the United States of America, 75 9, 4538-42 .

In 1976, Ewan Cameron and Linus Pauling published a study conducted on 100 cancer patients treated with vitamin C (10 grams of vitamin C via intravenous infusion for 10 days, followed by 10 grams of oral vitamin C per day). Their disease progress was compared to 1000 similar patients (by age, type of cancer, clinical stage etc.) treated identically, but without additional vitamin C. The mean survival time was 4.2 times higher for people who received vitamin C (210 days) compared to the controls (50 days). For 90% of patients treated with vitamin C, the survival time was 3 times that for the controls, while for 10% even averaging more than 20 times that for the controls. In the above follow-up study, they found that patients treated with vitamin C (usually 10 g/day) have a mean survival time about 300 days greater than that of the controls. In addition, survival time greater than one year in this group concerned 22% of patients, whereas for the controls it was only 0.4%. These results were therefore very promising. Nevertheless, it is worth noting that this study was not well designed as, for example, the placebo group was missing. Hence, this publication of these great scientists is not sufficient evidence of vitamin C's effectiveness in treating cancer. Later in the book, however, there will be such evidence.

Murata A, Morishige F, Yamaguchi H. **Prolongation of survival times of terminal cancer patients by administration of large doses of ascorbate.** Int J Vitam Nutr Res Suppl. 1982;23:103-13. PMID: 6811475.

A few years later, after the Americans, a similar study was carried out by the Japanese. They administered vitamin C to terminally ill cancer patients at two hospitals in Japan. At the Fukuoka Torikai Hospital there were 99 patients with terminal cancer. For 44 low-ascorbate patients the average survival time was 43 days, while for 55 high-ascorbate patients it was 246 days. Similar effects were seen in 26 patients at the Kamioka Kozan Hospital. For 19 control patients the average survival time was 48 days, while for 6 high-ascorbate patients it was 115 days. One patient was still alive. The authors concluded that large doses of vitamin C not only extended survival time but also improved the quality of life.

Animal studies

Campbell EJ, Dachs GU. **Current limitations of murine models in oncology for Ascorbate research.** Front Oncol. 2014;4:282.

After administration of a high dose of vitamin C in the amount of 30 mg/mouse (equivalent to 1 g/kg), sarcoma 180 tumor growth was inhibited. Similarly, continuous intraperitoneal injection of vitamin C at 4 g/kg resulted in reduction in hormone-refractory prostate tumor volume and a decrease in metastatic lesions of over 50%. Nude mice with human pancreatic tumor xenografts were given 4 g/kg of vitamin C. These xenographs were found to be significantly smaller in these mice than in the untreated ones. Same dose in mouse pancreatic cancer xenografts was found to reduce tumor volume by 42%. In yet another study, treatment with lower doses of vitamin C (0.15 g/kg) showed a large reduction in the rate of tumor growth of human colorectal cancer xenografts.

Other very relevant studies

Sen, U., Shenoy P, S., & Bose, B. (2017). **Opposing effects of low versus high concentrations of water soluble vitamins/dietary ingredients Vitamin C and niacin on colon cancer stem cells (CSCs)**. Cell Biology International, 41.

In this study, scientists investigated the effects of vitamin C and vitamin B3 on cancer stem cells (CSCs). CSCs are responsible for metastasis and relapses. As previous studies have shown, vitamin C in high doses selectively kills colon cancer cells having BRAF and KRAS mutations through the induced oxidative stress. It is important to add that BRAF and KRAS mutations occur in about 10% and about 44% of patients with metastatic colorectal cancer, respectively. In the above study, the results were similar, but depending on the concentration. Low concentrations of 5, 10, 15, 20 and 25 µM increased colon CSCs proliferation (an increase in the number of cancer cells as a result of cell growth), while high concentrations of 100 µM to 1000 µM exhibited a cell killing effect on colon cancer stem cells. Ultimately, the death effects of the study on CSCs were 50-60% and about 30% for HT-29 and HCT-15 colorectal carcinoma cell lines, respectively.

It is worth mentioning that vitamin C behaves in a similar way also in the case of skin cancer. Lower concentrations are associated with an increase in the melanoma growth, whereas higher concentrations (5 mM) significantly reduce cancer invasiveness.

Sant, David W et al. **"Vitamin C promotes apoptosis in breast cancer cells by increasing TRAIL expression."** Scientific Reports 8 (2018): n. pag.

Loss of 5hmC is common across many types of cancer. For instance, reduced levels of this important epigenetic mark that regulates gene expression is correlated with poorer survival in glioma. As it turned out, vitamin C was found to increase 5hmC content in breast cancer cells. Furthermore, vitamin C also induced apoptosis (programmed cancer cell death) in the same cells. Results, therefore suggested a potential role of vitamin C in breast cancer prevention and treatment.

Studies in mice that could not produce vitamin C and had melanoma or breast cancer showed that supplementation with this vitamin hindered metastasis, inflammatory cytokine secretion, and led to less tumor growth. Another study, in turn, indicated that high dose vitamin C (concentration of 2 mM) could stop migration and invasion of breast cancer cell lines by suppressing the epithelial – mesenchymal transition (EMT).

Seo, Min-Seok et al. **"High-Dose Vitamin C Promotes Regression of Multiple Pulmonary Metastases Originating from Hepatocellular Carcinoma."** Yonsei Medical Journal 56 (2015): 1449 - 1452.

I will also describe two of the many documented cases of the very beneficial effects of vitamin C in cancer. In this case, it concerns regression of multiple pulmonary metastases, which originated from hepatocellular carcinoma. A 74-year-old woman was admitted to the clinic for cancer-specific symptoms such as general weakness and anorexia. After undergoing initial transarterial chemoembolization (TACE), the doctors found local recurrence with multiple pulmonary metastases. The woman decided to refuse further conventional therapy. However, she opted for vitamin C. Consequently, she received 70 grams of intravenous vitamin C administered into a peripheral vein twice a week for 10 months. As it turned out, there was a complete regression of multiple pulmonary metastases.

Baillie, N., Carr, A.C., & Peng, S. (2018). **The Use of Intravenous Vitamin C as a Supportive Therapy for a Patient with Glioblastoma Multiforme.** Antioxidants, 7.

Another case was a 55-year-old woman with glioblastoma multiforme (high grade malignant brain tumor with median survival 12 months and 2% survival for three years). She was diagnosed in November 2010 with glioblastoma multiforme following a 10 days history of headaches and constipation. She underwent craniotomy and debulking surgery in December 2010, followed by a course of radiotherapy and temozolomide. The woman started vitamin C therapy three weeks after brain surgery. The patient received 85 grams of intravenous vitamin C three times a week for the first six months and then twice a week for over three years. After IV vitamin C treatments (January 2011) the patient reported improvement. She experienced improved energy and walking distance (prior to starting the first course of radiation therapy). The woman also continued vitamin C therapy during chemotherapy and radiotherapy, which she tolerated "pretty well". Additionally "Compared to the patient's QoL (health-related quality of life) data prior to commencing IV vitamin C treatment, dramatic improvement was reported in the three months survey following initiation of IV vitamin C treatment (at that time the patient had just completed radiotherapy and started chemotherapy) and the improvement was maintained for the first 12 months. Clinical symptoms such as fatigue, dyspnoea, insomnia, appetite loss and diarrhea resolved and the patient's physical and role functioning increased significantly, as well as 'global health status', which improved from 'very poor' to 'excellent'". In November 2014 her condition deteriorated and continued to deteriorate until 26 February 2015 when she passed away at home. The patient stopped getting intravenous vitamin C three months before her death.

Harris, H. R., Orsini, N. & Wolk, A. **Vitamin C and survival among women with breast cancer: a meta-analysis.** *Eur J Cancer.* 50, 1223–31 (2014).

The authors of this meta-analysis wanted to investigate the relationship between vitamin C and survival among women with breast cancer. In this regard, they analyzed several studies that examined vitamin C supplement use and dietary vitamin C intake, including 17,696 breast cancer cases, 2791 total deaths, and 1558 breast cancer-specific deaths. They found that the overall and breast cancer-specific risk of death for those who supplemented with vitamin C after diagnosis was reduced by 19% and 15%, respectively. Moreover, increasing vitamin C intake by 100 mg per day resulted in a risk reduction of 27% for total mortality and 22% for breast cancer-specific mortality.

Ma, Yan et al. **"High-Dose Parenteral Ascorbate Enhanced Chemosensitivity of Ovarian Cancer and Reduced Toxicity of Chemotherapy."** Science Translational Medicine 6 (2014): 222ra18 - 222ra18.

This randomized controlled trial involving patients diagnosed with stage III and stage IV ovarian cancer examined the effect of intravenous vitamin C on median overall survival. 13 patients were given 15-100 grams intravenous vitamin C twice a week plus chemotherapy treatment of carboplatin and paclitaxel. A control group of 12 patients received chemotherapy alone. Compared with participants treated with chemotherapy only, participants treated also with vitamin C had decreases in almost all the categories of toxicity, including neurotoxicity, bone marrow toxicity, infection, hepatobiliary/pancreatic toxicity, toxicities in the renal/genitourinary, pulmonary, and gastrointestinal systems, and dermatology. As it turned out, the median time for disease progression/relapse was 8.75 months longer for patients taking chemotherapy with vitamin C compared to the control group.

Günes-Bayir, A., & Kiziltan, H.S. (2015). **Palliative Vitamin C Application in Patients with Radiotherapy-Resistant Bone Metastases**: A Retrospective Study. Nutrition and Cancer, 67, 921 -925.

The authors of this study investigated the effect of vitamin C infusion on pain, performance status, and survival time in cancer patients with bone metastases treated with radiotherapy. Out of 39 patients, 15 people received chemotherapy, another 15 people received vitamin C infusion (2.5 g) and 9 people received neither chemotherapy nor this vitamin. In the group with vitamin C, 4 people (26%) had an increased performance status, in the group with chemotherapy it was 1 person, whereas in the control group there was no one. In the vitamin C group also, the median pain reduction was 50%. Moreover, the median survival time for people receiving vitamin C was 10 months, while in the control and chemotherapy groups this median was only 2 months.

Mikirova, Nina A. et al. **"Effect of high-dose intravenous vitamin C on inflammation in cancer patients."** Journal of Translational Medicine 10 (2012): 189 - 189.

As there is an association between inflammation and poor prognosis in many types of cancer, doctors at the Riordan Clinic decided to examine the effect of high doses of intravenous vitamin C therapy on inflammation in cancer patients. 45 patients with prostate cancer, breast cancer, bladder cancer, pancreatic cancer, lung cancer, thyroid cancer, skin cancer and B-cell lymphoma got vitamin C in a dose of 7.5 to 50 grams after standard treatments by conventional methods. CRP and tumor markers were measured routinely. After the intervention, a positive response to treatment was found in 75% of patients. The poorest response was related to aggressive stage cancer patients. However, as it turned out, inflammation cytokines IL-1α, IL-2, IL-8, TNF-α, chemokine eotaxin and CRP were reduced significantly after treatments with intravenous vitamin C. These results therefore indicated that intravenous high-dose vitamin C may significantly reduce inflammation in cancer patients.

Several different studies have confirmed that high-dose vitamin C can enhance the anti-cancer effects of such medications as doxorubicin, eribulin mesylate, tamoxifen, fulvestrant and trastuzumab. Additionally, studies have reported that 4g/kg intraperitoneal injection of vitamin C twice daily with gemcitabine can lead to significant tumor growth inhibition in pancreatic cancer, and the same dose of vitamin C with cisplatin enhances the therapeutic effect in oral squamous carcinoma.

Blaszczak, Wiktoria et al. **"Vitamin C as a Modulator of the Response to Cancer Therapy."** Molecules 24 (2019): n. pag.

Polish scientists in this publication indicated that high-dose vitamin C administration amongst patients with cancer can increase the quality of life, improve the physical and mental conditions and decrease adverse effects of chemotherapy. They concluded that high doses of vitamin C alone or in combination with standard cancer drugs significantly enhances suppression of tumor growth. These benefits result from both mechanisms dependent and independent from drugs. Importantly, they also noted that therapeutic plasma vitamin C levels are easily achieved only by intravenous administration.

Yeom, Chang Hwan et al. **"Changes of Terminal Cancer Patients' Health-related Quality of Life after High Dose Vitamin C Administration."** Journal of Korean Medical Science 22 (2007): 7 - 11.

These scientists wanted to investigate the effects of vitamin C on cancer patients' health-related quality of life. For this purpose, 39 terminal cancer patients were given an intravenous administration of 10 grams vitamin C twice with a 3-day interval and an oral intake of 4 g vitamin C daily for a week. Following intravenous vitamin C treatment, the patients reported significantly higher scores for physical, role, emotional, and cognitive function in the functional scale. In the case of symptom scale, the patients reported significantly lower scores for fatigue, nausea, vomiting, pain, and appetite loss. Overall, vitamin C has proven to be a cheap and effective method of improving the quality of life of terminal cancer patients.

Carr, A.C., & McCall, C. (2017). **The role of vitamin C in the treatment of pain:** new insights. Journal of Translational Medicine, 15.

Moreover vitamin C appears to be an effective adjunctive therapy for acute and chronic pain relief in many conditions. Such an effect of this vitamin, for example, as studies have shown, concerns the chronic regional pain syndrome. A similar effect applies to acute herpetic and postherpetic neuralgia, when vitamin C reduces symptoms. What interests us now, vitamin C in high doses also reduces cancer-related pain. This, of course, has a positive effect on patient quality of life.

Mansoor, Farah et al. **"Impact of Intravenous Vitamin C Administration in Reducing Severity of Symptoms in Breast Cancer Patients During Treatment."** Cureus 13 (2021): n. pag.

Let this research from 2021 be another good confirmation of what I wrote about above. 350 people with breast cancer participated in this single-center, parallel-group, single-blind interventional study were divided into two groups at a ratio of 1:1. One group was given 25 grams of vitamin C intravenously per week for four weeks in addition to their current standard treatment, while the other group was given only a placebo and their current standard treatment. Intravenous vitamin C has been shown to significantly reduce the mean severity score for symptoms such as nausea, loss of appetite, tumor pain, fatigue and insomnia.

NOTE: Despite the fact that intravenous administration of high amounts of vitamin C appears to be safe and adverse events are rare, there are a few things that require caution before starting therapy. These include, for example, renal insufficiency and red cell glucose-6-phosphate dehydrogenase deficiency (G6PD). High doses of vitamin C can also lead to a decrease in potassium levels, which, however, can be reversed by supplementing with this mineral. More on the potential side effects later.

Böttger, F., Vallés-Martí, A., Cahn, L. et al. **High-dose intravenous vitamin C, a promising multi-targeting agent in the treatment of cancer.** J Exp Clin Cancer Res 40, 343 (2021). https://doi.org/10.1186/s13046-021-02134-y

The authors of the above review of dozens of studies from October 2021 have summarized everything I wrote about in this chapter and come to following conclusions about vitamin C in cancer:

1. The anti-cancer effects can only be achieved through the intravenous administration of vitamin C.

2. For monotherapy, the effective dose of intravenous vitamin C ranges from 1.5g/kg to 1.9-2.2g/kg, while in combination from 75 g to 87.5 g in total will be sufficient.

3. Intravenous vitamin C should be administered at least twice a week. In studies showing high effectiveness, vitamin C was administered 2-3 times a week for at least 8 weeks.

In the words of the authors of this publication themselves: "To conclude, a large body of evidence is accumulating suggesting that VitC, when administered intravenously and in high doses, has potent cancer-selective cytotoxic, cancer-therapy sensitizing and toxicity-reducing properties."

Although we do not yet have a sufficient amount of studies involving liposomal vitamin C in cancer, we can assume that vitamin C given in this form may be an alternative, to some extent, to intravenous infusions. As I will prove in a moment, oral liposomal vitamin C in large amounts may result in plasma levels even above 400 µm (impossible to obtain with normal ascorbic acid taken orally). Regarding, for example, colon cancer, these are strongly anti-cancer levels.

CHAPTER 46: ORAL VS LIPOSOMAL VS INTRAVENOUS

This is a good time to describe these three ways to use vitamin C. This will help to understand, for example, why vitamin C given intravenously or even in a liposomal form in cancer will be better than oral vitamin C. And why in acute and severe cases, overall, intravenous vitamin C is usually the better choice. We will start with oral vitamin C.

The bioavailability of oral vitamin C is variable. This variability is mainly dependent on the dose and the frequency of administration. The maximum single dose that will not result in some vitamin C excretion in the urine seems to be approximately 200 mg. At higher doses, bioavailability decreases, and excess vitamin C is excreted in the urine. Some might think that we can now move on to intravenous vitamin C then. However, just because some of the vitamin C is excreted, it doesn't mean that the levels at higher doses do not increase further. And it is so.

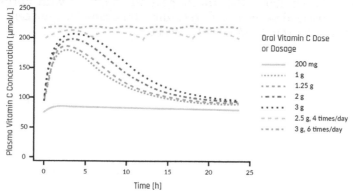

Oral Vitamin C Dose or Dosage

———	200 mg
··········	1 g
– · – · –	1.25 g
ı — — ı	2 g
· · · · ·	3 g
– – – –	2.5 g, 4 times/day
– · · – · ·	3 g, 6 times/day

Our 200 mg dose of vitamin C raises plasma vitamin C concentration to around 70-80 µmol/L. However, 3 grams of vitamin C can increase the concentration by up to three times to about 200 µmol/L. If this dose is maintained by giving several such doses, the peak plasma vitamin C concentration of 220 µmol/l may be also maintained. Of course, this does not mean that doses above these illustrative 3 grams make no therapeutic sense. You will find out about it later in this book.

Carr, Anitra C. et al. **"Human skeletal muscle ascorbate is highly responsive to changes in vitamin C intake and plasma concentrations123."** The American Journal of Clinical Nutrition 97 (2013): 800 - 807.

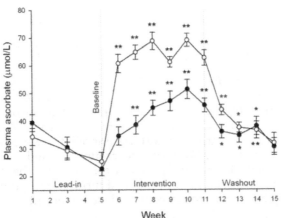

Importantly, the vitamin C level can also be raised to a decent level through food. Above, we can see plasma ascorbate concentrations in people who consumed 0.5 kiwifruit a day and 2 kiwifruits a day. At baseline in the low-kiwifruit dose group, the mean vitamin C level was 22.7 µmol/l, rising to a level of 45.5 µmol/l at the time of the intervention. In the high-kiwifruit dose group, this level increased from an initial 25.4 µmol/l to 62.6 µmol/l at the time of the intervention.

In the case of intravenous vitamin C, the situation is quite different. Here, the concentration of vitamin C can be even several dozen times higher than in the case of an oral vitamin. At these levels, we are already talking about millimoles per liter (1 mmol/l (mM) = 1000 μmol/l (μM)). The following graph illustrates this.

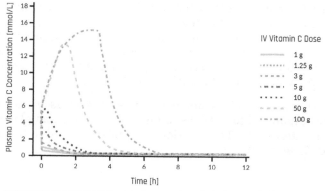

Predicted plasma vitamin C concentrations in healthy persons after oral (top) or intravenous (IV) (bottom) administration of vitamin C.

Adapted from: Padayatty, S.J.; Sun, H.; Wang, Y.; Riordan, H.D.; Hewitt, S.M.; Katz, A.; Wesley, R. A.; Levine, M. "Vitamin C Pharmacokinetics: Implications for Oral and Intravenous Use" *Ann Intern Med.* 2004;140(7):533-537. doi: 10.7326/0003-4819-140-7-200404060-00010

As you can see, our 3 grams of vitamin C given intravenously can increase the concentration to as much as 1800 μmol/L as opposed to 200 μmol/L when taken orally. 10 grams of vitamin C will be able to raise the concentration to about 6 mmol/l (6000 μmol/l). In turn, 50 and 100 grams of intravenous vitamin C will raise the concentration to around 14 and 16 mmol/L, respectively. Interestingly, as you can also see, the decrease in the concentration of both oral and intravenous vitamin C is relatively fast. This is why frequency is so important.

Liposomal vitamin C (i.e. vitamin C encapsulated in a lipid sphere) is also worth attention. As I already mentioned, the concentrations achieved with the oral use of liposomal vitamin C can exceed those concentrations achieved with the usual oral vitamin C. This matters and affects the effectiveness of the therapy. Nonetheless, it should be remembered that one liposomal vitamin C is not equal to the other liposomal vitamin C. Depending on the quality, different results can be expected.

Hickey, Stephen & Roberts, Hilary & Nicholas, & Miller, J. (2009). **Pharmacokinetics of oral vitamin C**. Journal of Nutritional and Environmental Medicine. 17. 10.1080/13590840802305423.

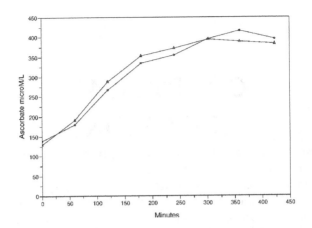

In this study, patients received 5 grams of oral vitamin C as well as 5, 20 and 36 grams of liposomal vitamin C. After consuming 5 grams of oral vitamin C, the concentration rose even just over 220 μmol/l. When 20 grams of liposomal vitamin C was administered, the concentration increased to approx. 330 μmol/l. In turn, when the patient was given 36 grams of liposomal vitamin C, the concentration, as seen above, increased to over 400 μmol/l.

CHAPTER 47:
INFECTIONS

Vitamin C is essential for the proper functioning of the immune system. It is important in prevention as well as extremely effective in treatment. Vitamin C is, above all, a potent antioxidant, i.e. it has the ability to donate electrons. In turn, all infections are associated with the excessive production of free radicals (molecules with unpaired electrons), which cause a lot of damage to the body. Vitamin C is able to neutralize these free radicals and protect the body from oxidative stress. Vitamin C supports epithelial barrier function against pathogens. Vitamin C, by accumulation in phagocytic cells, can enhance phagocytosis, chemotaxis and generation of reactive oxygen species, which will consequently increase the ability to kill microbes. Moreover, in lymphocytes, vitamin C enhances differentiation and proliferation of B- and T-cells (both responsible for adaptive immune response). When this vitamin is deficient, the immune system cannot function properly and is very susceptible to infection. What's more, once there is an infection, it can increase this vitamin C deficiency even more. This is very important so I'll repeat in other words; during an infection, the body's need for vitamin C may be even several times higher. Hence, usually high doses are most effective. This will also be shown in this chapter. We'll start with the common cold and end with sepsis. In addition, I will present the medical experience of two great doctors; Dr. Frederick R. Klenner and Dr. Robert F. Cathcart.

Cheng LL, Liu YY, Li B, Li SY, Ran PX. [**An in vitro study on the pharmacological ascorbate treatment of influenza virus**]. Zhonghua Jie He He Hu Xi Za Zhi. 2012 Jul;35(7):520-3. Chinese. PMID: 22931805.

The authors of this publication investigated the effects of pharmacological ascorbate against Influenza. They found that vitamin C concentration of 2.5 mmol/l was able to eliminate 90% of the viruses. Additionally, a much higher concentration (20 mmol/L) totally blocked viral replication in vitro.

Similarly, other studies have shown that, for example, vitamin C is able to decrease reverse transcriptase activity (used to replicate own genomes) by 99 percent of the virus type 1-infected cells.

Common cold

Hemilä, H. (1999). **Vitamin C supplementation and common cold symptoms: factors affecting the magnitude of the benefit**. Medical hypotheses, 52 2, 171-8 .

In this meta-analysis, the researchers analyzed 23 studies with regular vitamin C supplementation equal to or greater than 1 g/day. Vitamin C was, on average, more effective in children than in adults. In addition, a dose of vitamin C greater than or equal to 2 grams was more effective than that of 1 gram. The duration of colds decreased by 21% among adults taking 2 grams of vitamin C daily and by 6% among adults taking only 1 gram daily. The reduction in the duration of colds was even greater in children. Those children who took 2 grams of vitamin C per day had a 26% reduction in the duration of the common cold, whereas children who took only 1 gram of vitamin C 17%. It can be assumed that the fact that one dose (e.g. 2 grams) contributed to a greater reduction in the duration of colds in children than in adults is due to the fact that the child is simply smaller and these 2 grams correspond to a lower body weight than that of an adult. If adults took 3 or 4 grams of vitamin C, the results might be similar.

Ran, Li et al. **"Extra Dose of Vitamin C Based on a Daily Supplementation Shortens the Common Cold:** A Meta-Analysis of 9 Randomized Controlled Trials." BioMed Research International 2018 (2018): n. pag.

The authors of this meta-analysis of 9 studies wanted to investigate whether vitamin C is effective in the treatment of the common cold as a prophylactic measure with or without therapeutic doses of this vitamin taken after the onset of symptoms. Prophylactic doses ranged from 1-3 grams per day along with a therapeutic dose of up to 6 grams at the onset of symptoms. The authors found that prophylactic supplementation of vitamin C along with a therapeutic dose at the onset of common cold symptoms is capable of relieving chest pain, fever, and chills and reduce the duration of a cold episode. Only the therapeutic dose given at the onset of symptoms did not produce such effects. In turn, prophylactic taking of vitamin C and then administration of extra doses of vitamin C at the onset of a common cold could help reduce the duration by about half a day.

Douglas, R.M., & Hemilä, H. (2005). **Vitamin C for Preventing and Treating the Common Cold**. PLoS Medicine, 2.

These scientists investigated whether vitamin C used either as continuous prophylaxis or after the onset of cold symptoms can reduce incidence, duration or severity of the common cold. Doses in the studies were 200 mg and above. A subgroup of six trials involving a total of 642 marathon runners, skiers, and soldiers reported vitamin C resulted in 50% fewer colds. Moreover, based on thirty comparisons that involved 9,676 respiratory episodes, it was concluded that supplementation led to an 8% reduction in cold duration for adults and a 13.5% reduction for children.

Kim, Tae kyung et al. **"Vitamin C supplementation reduces the odds of developing a common cold in Republic of Korea Army recruits: randomised controlled trial."** BMJ Military Health 168 (2020): 117 - 123.

This randomized, placebo-controlled, and double-blind trial aimed to investigate whether vitamin C intake can prevent common colds in Republic of Korea Army soldiers. 1444 participants were divided into two groups. 695 participants received 6 grams of vitamin C per day, while 749 participants received a placebo. As it turned out, the vitamin C supplementation group had a 0.80-fold lower risk of getting a common cold than did the placebo group. Additionally, subgroup analysis showed that vitamin C was more effective among never smokers and among those in physical rank 3.

Respiratory infections

Gorton, H.C., & Jarvis, K.K. (1999). **The effectiveness of vitamin C in preventing and relieving the symptoms of virus-induced respiratory infections. Journal of manipulative and physiological therapeutics**, 22 8, 530-3 .

In this study, scientists investigated the effectiveness of vitamin C in preventing and relieving the symptoms of respiratory infections. To this end, 463 students aged 18 to 32 years were included in the control group and 252 students aged 18 to 30 years in the experimental or test group. Investigators tracked the number of reports of cold and flu symptoms in both the control group and the test group. When symptoms appeared in the control group, the subjects were treated with pain relievers and decongestants. In contrast, people in the test group received 1 gram of vitamin C every hour for 6 hours and then 3 times a day when they got symptoms. Additionally, people in the test group were given 1 gram of vitamin C three times a day if they were not reporting symptoms. The results were as follows: "Overall, reported flu and cold symptoms in the test group decreased 85% compared with the control group after the administration of megadose Vitamin C."

Hemilä, H., & Chalker, E. (2019). **Vitamin C Can Shorten the Length of Stay in the ICU**: A Meta-Analysis. Nutrients, 11.

The authors of this meta-analysis wanted to evaluate whether vitamin C has an effect on length of stay in the intensive care unit (ICU) and duration of mechanical ventilation. They analyzed 18 relevant controlled trials with a total of 2004 patients. They found that in 12 trials with 1766 patients, vitamin C reduced the length of ICU stay on average by nearly 8%. In six trials, orally administered vitamin C in doses from 1 to 3 grams per day reduced the length of ICU stay by 8.6%. In addition, vitamin C shortened the duration of mechanical ventilation by 18.2% in patients who required mechanical ventilation for over 24 hours.

Hemilä, H., & Chalker, E. (2020). **Vitamin C may reduce the duration of mechanical ventilation in critically ill patients: a meta-regression analysis.** Journal of Intensive Care, 8.

The authors of the previous meta-analysis that indicated that vitamin C may shorten the length of ICU stay also analyzed studies suggesting vitamin C effect on ventilation time. Hence this meta-analysis was created, covering 8 studies and 685 patients in total. The pooled result indicated that vitamin C could reduce the length of mechanical ventilation by an average of 14%. However, there was a large heterogeneity in the results. The higher the dose, the better the results usually. Based on an analysis of five studies including 471 patients requiring ventilation for over 10 hours, vitamin C in amounts ranging from 1 to 6 grams per day shortened ventilation time on average by 25%. Overall, vitamin C administration has been most beneficial to patients with the longest ventilation (i.e. the most severely ill).

Hemilä H, Douglas RM. **Vitamin C and acute respiratory infections**. Int J Tuberc Lung Dis. 1999 Sep;3(9):756-61. PMID: 10488881.

Hemilä and Douglas in this study have reviewed many publications about the effects of vitamin C on infections. They pointed out that in four trials of British males common cold incidence decreased by on average 30% when study participants were getting vitamin C. In relation to this vitamin, in two of these studies absence from school and work was reduced by 14-21% per episode. Moreover, three controlled studies found a roughly 80% decrease in the incidence of pneumonia in participants who took vitamin C, compared to those who did not. One study also showed a significant positive effect of vitamin C in elderly UK patients hospitalized with pneumonia or bronchitis.

Hemilä H. **Vitamin C and Infections. Nutrients.** 2017 Mar 29;9(4):339. doi: 10.3390/nu9040339. PMID: 28353648; PMCID: PMC5409678.

Dr. Harri Hemilä wrote in this review covering evidence of vitamin C's effectiveness in preventing and treating infections: "Two controlled trials found a statistically significant dose-response, for the duration of common cold symptoms, with up to 6–8 g/day of vitamin C. Thus, the negative findings of some therapeutic common cold studies might be explained by the low doses of 3–4 g/day of vitamin C. Three controlled trials found that vitamin C prevented pneumonia. Two controlled trials found a treatment benefit of vitamin C for pneumonia patients. One controlled trial reported treatment benefits for tetanus patients." Dr. Hemilä stated that the best results appear when vitamin C treatment is started at the onset of symptoms. Moreover, vitamin C must be given regularly (multiple times per day) and in a dose of at least 6 grams or more.

Hunt C, Chakravorty NK, Annan G, Habibzadeh N, Schorah CJ. **The clinical effects of vitamin C supplementation in elderly hospitalised patients with acute respiratory infections.** Int J Vitam Nutr Res. 1994;64(3):212-9. PMID: 7814237.

In this randomized double-blind trial, researchers examined the effects of vitamin C on acute respiratory infections. The study was conducted on 57 elderly patients admitted to hospital with bronchitis, bronchopneumonia and vitamin C deficiencies (patients' blood vitamin C levels were 23 micromoles per liter). Patients were given either 200 mg of vitamin C per day or a placebo. As it turned out, even such a relatively small dose of vitamin C resulted in significant improvements in major respiratory functions. Perhaps it was associated with severe vitamin C deficiency in the treated patients.

A.A. Syed, S. Knowlson, R. Sculthorpe, et al. **Phase I safety trial of intravenous ascorbic acid in patients with severe sepsis** J Transl Med, 12 (2014), p. 32

The above study examined the effect of α-tocopherol (1000 IU) and ascorbate (1 g intravenously every 8 h for 28 days) in preventing the development of pulmonary morbidity (ARDS, pneumonia) and organ failure in severely ill surgical patients. The patients were divided into the group treated with antioxidants and receiving standard care. Scientists found 19% reduction in incidence of pulmonary morbidity in patients receiving antioxidants. In addition, the antioxidant treated group had a 57% lower incidence of multiple organ failure and a trend toward a reduction in 28-day mortality.

Fowler III, Alpha A et al. **"Intravenous vitamin C as adjunctive therapy for enterovirus/rhinovirus induced acute respiratory distress syndrome."** World Journal of Critical Care Medicine 6 (2017): 85 - 90.

It is also worth mentioning the case reported by dr. Alpha A. Fowler. This is a case of virus-induced acute respiratory distress syndrome (ARDS) treated with intravenous vitamin C. A 20 year old woman contracted respiratory enterovirus/rhinovirus infection. That resulted in acute lung injury and ARDS. Because support with mechanical ventilation failed, extracorporeal membrane oxygenation (ECMO) was initiated. At 12 hours following the initiation of ECMO, high-dose intravenous vitamin C was also started with a dose of 200 mg/kg every 24 hours divided equally into four doses. The patient improved rapidly. ECMO and mechanical ventilation were discontinued by day 7 and patient recovered with no evidence of post-ARDS fibroproliferative sequelae.

Other infections

González, Michael J. et al. "**High Dose Intravenous Vitamin C Treatment for Zika Fever**." (2016).

Another case report concerns a 54 year old woman with symptomatology congruent with Zika fever. Three days after several mosquito bites the woman noted the onset of fever and chills. Soon there was also a sore mouth and oral blisters developed. On the fifth day a papular rash appeared. Due to an ongoing rash, a retro-orbital headache, fever and significant joint and muscle tenderness, the woman went to the doctor. After testing positive for flaviviruses, the doctor began treatment with vitamin C. Vitamin C was applied in escalating doses of 25 grams (first day), 50 grams (second day) and 75 grams (third day). Symptoms improved significantly within 24 hours of starting therapy and were absent by the third day.

Chen, Shuangdi et al. "**Clinical Effect of Intravenous Vitamin C on Viral Myocarditis in Children: A Systematic Review and Meta-Analysis.**" Evidence-based Complementary and Alternative Medicine : eCAM 2019 (2019): n. pag.

The authors of this meta-analysis compared the effects of conventional therapy combined with intravenous vitamin C and conventional therapy alone on viral myocarditis in children. 426 children got conventional therapy and intravenous vitamin C in an amount ranging from 100 to 250 mg/kg, whereas 363 children (control group) received conventional therapy alone.

Compared to conventional treatment alone, such treatment, with the addition of vitamin C, resulted in better total effective rate and lower lactate dehydrogenase (LDH), creatine kinase (CK), and creatine kinase isoenzyme (CK-MB) levels (high levels of these enzymes are associated with myocardial ischemia and lesions).

Chen, Jen-Yin et al. **"Plasma Vitamin C Is Lower in Postherpetic Neuralgia Patients and Administration of Vitamin C Reduces Spontaneous Pain but Not Brush-evoked Pain."** The Clinical Journal of Pain 25 (2009): 562-569.

Postherpetic neuralgia (PHN) is a long-term nerve pain and a complication of shingles. The authors of this publication conducted two studies related to this ailment. The first study included 39 healthy volunteers and 38 PHN patients in whom plasma concentrations of vitamin C were measured. These plasma concentrations in patients with PHN were found to be significantly lower than in healthy volunteers (by approximately 66%). The second study was a double-blinded, placebo-controlled intervention study that enrolled 41 patients and divided them into an ascorbate group and a placebo. The ascorbate group got 2.5 grams of intravenous vitamin C on days 1, 3, and 5. As it turned out, patients who received the infusions reported having less pain compared to the control group.

Mikirova N, Hunninghake R. **Effect of high dose vitamin C on Epstein-Barr viral infection.** Med Sci Monit. 2014 May 3;20:725-32. doi: 10.12659/MSM.890423. PMID: 24793092; PMCID: PMC4015650.

Nina Mikirova and Ronald Hunninghake examined the effect of intravenous vitamin C on patients with Epstein-Barr virus (EBV) infection. 178 patients showed elevated levels of EBV EA IgG and 40 showed elevated levels of EBV VCA IgM (these are antibodies that indicate an infection). They received 7.5 to 50 grams of intravenous vitamin C. The decrease in antibodies amounted to 46% for subjects treated more than five times with intravenous vitamin C.

Jahan K, Ahmad K, Ali MA. **Effect of ascorbic acid in the treatment of tetanus.** Bangladesh Med Res Counc Bull. 1984 Jun;10(1):24-8. PMID: 6466264.

In this study, Dr. Jahan reported the effects of intravenous vitamin C in tetanus patients aged 1-30 years. Patients received 1 gram of intravenous vitamin C along with standard treatment (anti tetanus serum, sedatives and antibiotics) or standard treatment only. As it turned out, none of the 31 children (aged 1-12) died in the group treated with vitamin C and conventional medications. On the other hand, as many as 74.2% of tetanus children in the control group (n = 31) died. In the group of 27 older patients (aged 13-30) treated with vitamin C and standard drugs, the mortality was 37%. On the other hand, in the group of 38 patients not treated with vitamin C, the mortality rate was 67.8%. It is worth noting that vitamin C was administered in the same dose, regardless of age. And consequently the children got relatively more of this vitamin (per kg of body weight). This is perhaps why the mortality in group 1-12 was significantly lower than in group 13-30.

Schencking, M. Schulze et al. **"Intravenous Vitamin C in the treatment of shingles: Results of a multicenter prospective cohort study."** Medical Science Monitor : International Medical Journal of Experimental and Clinical Research 18 (2012): CR215 - CR224.

Schencking and Schulze examined the effects of intravenous vitamin C in patients with shingles. 67 participants with symptomatic herpes zoster were included in this study. The patients were subsequently administered 7.5 g intravenous vitamin C two to four times a week for a total of 2 weeks. 35.3% of the patients received no other drug therapies for herpes zoster. The assessment of pain (10-point VAS) was measured at baseline, after 2 weeks and after 12 weeks. Baseline mean pain was 5.8. After two weeks, the VAS was 2.2, whereas after 12 weeks it was only 0.6. Overall, 92% of patients experienced pain reduction after treatment. Despite the lack of a control group, the results seemed to be promising.

COVID-19

Tomasa-Irriguible, T.M., Bielsa-Berrocal, L. **COVID-19: Up to 82% critically ill patients had low Vitamin C values**. Nutr J 20, 66 (2021). https://doi.org/10.1186/s12937-021-00727-z

As we know, in the case of a large number of ailments, the level of vitamin C is significantly lowered. The authors of this publication proved that this also applies to COVID-19. They measured plasma vitamin C levels in critically ill COVID-19 adult patients who met acute respiratory distress syndrome (ARDS) criteria. They found that 82% of patients had low vitamin C values. Moreover, for 18% of patients, vitamin C values were undetectable.

Xia, Guozhi et al. "**High-dose intravenous vitamin C attenuates hyperinflammation in severe coronavirus disease 2019.**" Nutrition (Burbank, Los Angeles County, Calif.) 91 (2021): 111405 - 111405.

The authors of this publication wanted to evaluate the effectiveness of high-dose intravenous vitamin C on hyperinflammation in patients with severe COVID-19. To this end, they enrolled 236 patients, of which 151 were not getting vitamin C and 85 were getting (100 mg/kg every 6 hours for one day and then 100 mg/kg every 12 hours for 5 days). Initially, increased levels of inflammatory markers such as high-sensitivity C-reactive protein (hs-CRP), interleukin-6 (IL-6), tumor necrosis factor-α (TNF-α) were found in 80.1%, 91.5% and 67.4%, respectively. As it turned out, intravenous vitamin C significantly decreased these inflammatory markers (hs-CRP, IL-6, TNF-α) compared to placebo, contributing to the attenuation of hyperinflammation.

Sepsis

Sepsis is defined as a widespread, severe inflammatory reaction of the entire body in response to infection. Most often, bacteria and the toxins they produce are responsible for the development of sepsis, although it can also be caused by parasites, fungi or viruses. For example, COVID-19 can also lead to this condition. Sepsis poses a direct threat to the patient's life as it is associated with a significant risk of developing multi-organ failure and septic shock, which in turn is often fatal. As I will prove in a moment, vitamin C can prevent this from happening. Studies have shown that vitamin C deficiency (i.e., <11 μmol/L) and hypovitaminosis C (i.e., <23 μmol/L) in septic shock patients may affect even 40% and 90%, respectively. However, it is the high doses that can be crucial in the treatment process.

Fisher, Bernard J et al. "**Attenuation of sepsis-induced organ injury in mice by vitamin C.**" JPEN. Journal of parenteral and enteral nutrition 38 7 (2014): 825-39.

In this study, scientists investigated the effects of vitamin C on sepsis-induced multiple organ dysfunction syndrome in mice. The study was conducted on vitamin C sufficient and vitamin C deficient mice (that could not produce vitamin C on their own). In these mice, sepsis was induced by an infusion of a fecal stem solution. Additionally, some of the vitamin C deficient mice received an infusion of ascorbic acid in the amount of 200 mg/kg. Multiple organ dysfunction syndrome occurred in vitamin C deficient mice. In turn, this syndrom was not evident in vitamin C sufficient mice and attenuated in vitamin C deficient mice infused with ascorbic acid. Any abnormalities also in the coagulation system and circulating blood cells were attenuated by vitamin C.

Fowler, Alpha A Berry et al. "**Effect of Vitamin C Infusion on Organ Failure and Biomarkers of Inflammation and Vascular Injury in Patients With Sepsis and Severe Acute Respiratory Failure: The CITRIS-ALI Randomized Clinical Trial.**" JAMA 322 13 (2019): 1261-1270.

This is the first randomized clinical trial that investigated the effects of moderate dosages of intravenous vitamin C on patients with sepsis and severe acute respiratory failure (ARDS). 167 enrolled patients were divided into two groups. 84 people in the first group were administered intravenous vitamin C in the amount of 50 mg/kg every 6 hours for 96 hour and 83 patients in the second group were given a placebo. As it turned out, scientists could not detect any significant differences in the primary endpoint outcomes between the vitamin C and placebo group. Primary endpoints included Sequential Organ Failure Assessment (SOFA) score, C-reactive protein levels and thrombomodulin levels. However, in the case of secondary endpoint outcomes, there were significant differences. They concerned: 28-day mortality, Kaplan-Meier survival curves, ventilator-free days, ICU-free days, transfer out of the ICU by hour 168 and hospital free days. At day 28, mortality was 46.3% in the placebo group and 29.8% in the vitamin C group. However, within 96 hours (i.e. when one group was still receiving vitamin C), 4 people in the vitamin C group died, whereas 19 people in the placebo group died. The number of ventilator-free days for the vitamin C group was 13.1 and for the placebo group 10.6. Furthermore, the number of ICU-free days to day 28 was 10.7 in the vitamin C group and 7.7 in the placebo group. The transfer out of the ICU up to 168 hours concerned 25% of people in the vitamin C group and 12.5% of people in the placebo group. Finally, the number of hospital free days was 22.6 for the vitamin C group and 15.5 for the placebo group.

Fowler, Alpha A Berry et al. "**Phase I safety trial of intravenous ascorbic acid in patients with severe sepsis.**" Journal of Translational Medicine 12 (2013): 32 - 32.

The same author several years ago conducted a smaller randomized, double-blind, placebo-controlled trial on patients with severe sepsis (septic shock). Twenty-four patients in the medical intensive care unit were randomized 1:1:1. One group received intravenous vitamin C 50 mg/kg/day, the second group 200 mg/kg/day and the third placebo. Patients receiving intravenous vitamin C had reductions in SOFA scores compared to placebo. In addition, vitamin C significantly reduced the proinflammatory biomarkers C-reactive protein and procalcitonin (used often as a marker for the diagnosis of bacterial infections). Unlike the placebo group, also thrombomodulin in patients with vitamin C exhibited no significant rise.

Zabet MH, Mohammadi M, Ramezani M, Khalili H. **Effect of high-dose Ascorbic acid on vasopressor's requirement in septic shock.** J Res Pharm Pract 2016;5:94-100

These researchers wanted to investigate the effect of vitamin C on various parameters of septic shock in nonsurgical critically ill patients. Patients received a vasopressor drug to maintain mean arterial pressure over 65 mmHg as well as vitamin C in the amount of 100 mg/kg/day for three days or a placebo. As it turned out, people in the group with vitamin C needed much less of this drug. Moreover, 28-day mortality was 14.28% in the vitamin C group and 64.28% in the placebo group.

Marik PE, et al. **"Hydrocortisone, Vitamin C, and Thiamine for the Treatment of Severe Sepsis and Septic Shock A Retrospective Before-After Study"**. Chest. 2017. 151(6):1229-1238.

In this retrospective before-after clinical study researchers compared the outcome and clinical course of septic patients treated with intravenous vitamin C, hydrocortisone, and thiamine with outcome of control group treated in ICU. For the treatment group the hospital mortality was 8.5%, whereas for the placebo group over 40%. The aforementioned Sepsis-Related Organ Failure Assessment (SOFA) score decreased in all patients in the treatment group. Moreover, all patients in the treatment group have stopped requiring vasopressors. The mean duration of use of these drugs in the treatment group was 18.3 hours, whereas in the placebo group it was 54.9 hours.

In the last few years, there have also been several other studies showing the effectiveness of vitamin C therapy in combination with thiamine and hydrocortisone (HAT therapy).

Dr. Frederick Klenner

Dr. Frederick Klenner (1907-1984) was one of the pioneers in the use of vitamin C. Already in the 1940s, he published his first paper on vitamin C and the treatment of viral diseases. Over the next forty years he treated various diseases and conditions with vitamin C, including pneumonia, poliomyelitis, hepatitis, herpes simplex, chicken pox, measles, mumps, mononucleosis, pancreatitis, rheumatic fever, tetanus, cancer, arthritis, diabetes, schizophrenia, heavy metal poisonings and Black Widow Spider poisoning. Here, I would like to present a few cases from his medical practice.

Clinical Guide to the Use of Vitamin C, Lendon H. Smith. M.D, AscorbateWeb, 1988.

Viral pneumonia
A 28-year-old woman with a severe headache and stupor came to see the doctor. She was dehydrated and felt chest and head cold. Previous antibiotic treatment did not help. Dr. Klenner gave her 4 grams of vitamin C and 1000 cc of 5% dextrose. Within 11

hours her temperature dropped. Then, every two or three hours, she would get 2 to 4 grams of intravenous vitamin C. Within 72 hours, the woman's health improved significantly. For the next two weeks, she was getting 2 more grams of vitamin C every twelve hours. She was also given thiamine for deafness.

A 16 month old boy suddenly collapsed into unconsciousness after having a mild cold for two weeks. His pulse was over 200, and respiration 40 per minute. The doctor gave oxygen as well as 2 grams of intramuscular vitamin C. The boy roused in ten minutes. Next, the doctor administered 2 grams every two hours five times and then every four hours twelve times. As the examination showed bilateral pneumonitis, the patient was also given achromycin (antibiotic). Temperature dropped to normal by the third day and the child came home by the end of the week.

Mumps
A 23 year old man came to the doctor with mumps plus bilateral orchitis. He had a fever and was in great pain. This pain began to subside after 1 gram of vitamin C intravenously. Also, after six such injections every two hours, the pain was completely gone. After 36 hours, the fever went down and he was well in 60 hours. The total dose needed for this was 25 grams.

Polio
Dr. Klenner is known to heal all 60 polio patients during the poliomyelitis epidemic. As for vitamin C, he recommended a dose of 300 to 500 mg/kg for this ailment, and for young children, 2-3 grams intramuscularly every two to four hours. Here are two clinical cases of the treatment of polio:
1. A five year-old girl with paralysis of both legs came to the doctor. She also suffered from knee and back pain. The girl received vitamin C injections and a massage. Within four days she could move both legs. Already at home, she continued the therapy by taking 1 gram of oral vitamin C every two hours. She walked by the eleventh day. After completing her vitamin C therapy, she began taking vitamin B1 (10 milligrams) four times a day. The girl completely recovered by the 19th day.
2. The next polio patient had a severe headache, red eyes, suffered from vomiting and felt tightness in the hamstrings. The doctor administered 2 grams of intravenous vitamin C immediately and

again in two hours. The patient then received this dose every four hours for 48 hours. Six hours after starting treatment, the temperature dropped and the patient was able to sit and drink fluids. The patient then took 1.5 grams of vitamin C every two hours for a week and then started supplementing with vitamin B1.

Hepatitis

A 27-year-old man had jaundice, nausea and elevated temperature. He was given 60 grams of sodium ascorbate intravenously. Additionally, he got 5 grams of vitamin C orally every four hours. Three hours after the first intravenous injection, he was given 15 grams of vitamin C. Subsequently, twelve hours after the start of treatment, he was given another 60 grams of vitamin C. And another 15 grams after two hours. In total, for 30 hours, he received 270 grams of intravenous vitamin C and 45 grams of oral vitamin C (without diarrhea). The man's temperature then was normal and urine was clear of bile. He was discharged from the hospital.

Another young man (22 years old) with chills, fever and diagnosed viral hepatitis was admitted (his roommate had been admitted one day earlier). The man was given 15 grams of intravenous vitamin C every twelve hours for three days and then once a day for six days. Additionally, he took 5 grams of sodium ascorbate every four hours. On the sixth day he was discharged from the hospital and had no fever as well as bile in the urine. His roommate was in the hospital for 26 days.

Dr. Klenner also presented the case of a man with chronic hepatitis who was unsuccessfully treated with steroids. Patient was given B-complex and sodium ascorbate 45 grams three times a week. The patient also took 5 grams of vitamin C every four hours. Within five months, he was completely disease free. Later, Dr. Klenner stated that if he had administered the higher doses more frequently in the hospital, he could have healed the patient in a few weeks.

Schizophrenia

In the case of schizophrenia, Dr.Klenner referred to the work of Dr. Abram Hoffer and Dr. Humphrey Osmond, who proposed high doses of niacin (3 to 18 grams/day) and vitamin C (3 grams/day) to treat this disease. He stated that 6 to 8 grams of vitamin C was needed for niacin to work, and he reported one case of a person who, taking one gram of vitamin C every hour for 48 hours, got rid of the disease for 6 months.

Pancreatitis
Dr. Klenner also reported one case of pancreatitis. The sick patient was administered 60 grams of sodium ascorbate intravenously. The patient was able to go home in twelve hours.

Dr. Robert Cathcart

Another doctor with remarkable clinical experience was Robert F. Cathcart (1932-2007). Dr. Cathcart treated more than 20,000 patients throughout his medical practice with high doses of vitamin C and very good results.

Cathcart, Robert F.. **"Vitamin C, titrating to bowel tolerance, anascorbemia, and acute induced scurvy."** Medical hypotheses 7 11 (1981): 1359-76 .

From the early 1970s until this publication was written, Dr. Robert F. Cathcart treated more than 9,000 patients with high doses of vitamin C. This doctor, in turn, preferred vitamin C given orally. Depending on the condition, the doses used varied as the patient needed different amounts of vitamin C. He argued that the best way to measure vitamin C requirement for the patient is through bowel tolerance (until vitamin C finally causes diarrhea). Importantly, he noticed that bowel tolerance during illness can be up to 10 times greater than when we are healthy. In other words, vitamin C tolerance increases in proportion to the severity of the disease. Dr. Cathcart claimed that the maximum relief of symptoms occurs when vitamin C almost starts to cause diarrhea ("almost" is an important word here). He called this process: titrating to bowel tolerance. Moreover, he said from his own experience that most people tolerate high doses of ascorbic acid well. Young people usually respond slightly better to this vitamin. Overall, however, high doses of oral vitamin C appear to be very safe. Dr. Cathcart also provided representative recovery doses for each condition:

CONDITION	GRAMS OF ASCORBIC ACID PER DAY	NUMBER OF DOSES PER DAY
mild cold	30 - 60	6 - 10
severe cold	60 - 100+	8 - 15
influenza	100 - 150	8 - 20
mononucleosis	150 - 200+	12 - 25
viral pneumonia	100 - 200+	12 - 25
hay fever, asthma	15 - 50	4 - 8
allergy	0.5 - 50	4 - 8
burn, injury, surgery	25 - 150+	6 - 20
anxiety, exercise	15 - 25	4 - 6
cancer	15 - 100	4 - 15
rheumatoid arthritis	15 - 100	4 - 15
bacterial infections	30 - 200+	10 - 25
infectious hepatitis	30 - 100	6 - 15
candidiasis	15 - 200+	6 - 25

CHAPTER 48:
ATHEROSCLEROSIS

Cardiovascular disease is the leading cause of death for men and women in the world. In the United States alone, one person dies from cardiovascular disease every about 30 seconds. Annually, it is almost 700,000 deaths in this country. Globally, there are over 17 million deaths from this disease every year. This terrible statistic forces doctors and scientists to look for the causes of this real epidemic. Some of them have concluded that one of these causes may be a vitamin C deficiency. This conclusion does not seem unfounded. Many studies have found that vitamin C may play a huge role in atherosclerosis. We will delve into this research. As this is a very serious problem in today's world, we will also try to do it profoundly. Initially, we will look at several studies, including mostly observational studies, investigating vitamin C intake and cardiovascular health. Later we will look at what role a vitamin C deficiency may play in initiating the disease. The last part, the longest, will concern the relationship between the well-known risk factors for atherosclerosis and vitamin C. Perhaps all people diagnosed with atherosclerosis who are concerned about whether they will get a heart attack or stroke tomorrow will start taking vitamin C after reading this chapter. Perhaps people who want to prevent atherosclerosis will reach for this vitamin as well. We'll see.

WILLIS GC, LIGHT AW, GOW WS. **Serial arteriography in atherosclerosis.** Can Med Assoc J. 1954 Dec;71(6):562-8. PMID: 13209447; PMCID: PMC1825016.

The first to show that atherosclerosis can be reversible was Dr. G.C. Willis, who as early as in 1954 conducted a study on the development of atherosclerosis examining the femoral and popliteal arteries. The subjects were getting 500 mg of ascorbic acid three times a day (a total of 1500 mg a day). After 2-6 months, arteriography was repeated using the same standard technique. Without treatment none of 6 patients improved. On the other hand, in the treated group 6 out of 10 patients improved. In conclusion, this angiography study showed that vitamin C could reduce atherosclerotic plaques in humans.

Dingchao, He et al. **"The protective effects of high-dose ascorbic acid on myocardium against reperfusion injury during and after cardiopulmonary bypass**." The Thoracic and cardiovascular surgeon 42 5 (1994): 276-8 .

This study, in turn, found the protective effect of high-dose ascorbic acid on the myocardium in 85 patients undergoing cardiopulmonary bypass. The dose was 250 mg/kg body weight, which means that the average dose was even over a dozen grams. In 12.5% of those untreated with vitamin C, defibrillation was required, while in the group with vitamin C, no one required it. The cardiac index (CI) measured in the group with vitamin C was higher than in the group without. Furthermore, patients who got vitamin C needed shorter intensive care unit and hospital stays than those who did not get vitamin C. The authors concluded: "The results indicate that ascorbic acid can act as a scavenger of free radicals to decrease the peroxidation of the lipids present in the cell membrane and remove the radicals to protect the myocardium from ischemia-reperfusion injury effectively during and after open-heart operation."

Tomoda, Haruo et al. **"Possible prevention of postangioplasty restenosis by ascorbic acid**." The American journal of cardiology 78 11 (1996): 1284-6 .

At this point, it is also worth mentioning one study related to angioplasty (a procedure of using a balloon to stretch open a narrowed or blocked artery) and vitamin C. The aim of the study was to investigate the effect of ascorbic acid on post angioplasty restenosis. The study found that the incidence of restenosis in 50 people who supplemented with 500 mg of ascorbic acid per day was significantly lower compared to the control group of 51 people. The result indicated, therefore, the attenuating effect of vitamin C on restenosis.

Enstrom, James E. et al. "**Vitamin C Intake and Mortality among a Sample of the United States Population.**" Epidemiology 3 (1992): 194-202.

Moving on to observational studies. The authors of this publication examined the relation between vitamin C intake and mortality in the First National Health and Nutrition Examination Survey (NHANES I). 11,348 adults aged 25-74 years were observed. The median follow-up was 10 years and 1,809 deaths were recorded during this time. Dietary intake as well as supplementation were taken into account. Scientists estimated that men who had the highest vitamin C intakes had a 42% lower risk of dying from cardiovascular disease. For women who consumed the highest amounts of vitamin C, the risk was 25% lower.

Osganian SK, Stampfer MJ, Rimm E, et al. **Vitamin C and risk of coronary heart disease in women.** J Am Coll Cardiol. 2003; 42(2):246–252.

Scientists examined the relation between vitamin C intake and risk of coronary heart disease (CHD) in women. Based on a detailed semiquantitative food-frequency questionnaire, they estimated consumption of vitamin C and other nutrients of 85,118 women. Subsequently nurses were followed up for 16 years for the development of incident CHD. During this time, there were 1,356 incident cases of CHD. Women in the highest quintile of vitamin C intakes from diet and supplements of over 360 mg/day had 27% lower risk of nonfatal myocardial infarction and fatal CHD than women in the lowest quintile of intake below 93 mg/day. Interestingly, the risk reduction only appeared to affect women supplementing vitamin C.

Knekt P, Ritz J, Pereira MA, et al. **Antioxidant vitamins and coronary heart disease risk: a pooled analysis of 9 cohorts.** Am J Clin Nutr. 2004; 80(6):1508–1520.

Knekt, et al, wanted to investigate the relation between the intake of antioxidant vitamins and coronary heart disease (CHD) risk. To this end, they analyzed 9 prospective studies that included information on intakes of vitamin E, carotenoids, and vitamin C. Among the 293 172 subjects there were 4,647 CHD events during a 10 years follow-up. It turned out that people who supplemented with vitamin C in an amount above 700 mg per day had a reduced risk of CHD by 25% compared with subjects who did not take supplemental vitamin C.

Deicher, Robert et al. **"Low total vitamin C plasma level is a risk factor for cardiovascular morbidity and mortality in hemodialysis patients."** Journal of the American Society of Nephrology : JASN 16 6 (2005): 1811-8 .

These scientists included 138 hemodialysis patients in the study, whose total plasma vitamin C levels were measured at the baseline. Patients were then followed for the occurrence of adverse cardiac events or death. Major adverse cardiovascular events (MACE) occurred in 35 patients (25%) over a period of median 30 months. In addition, 42 patients (30%) died (29 cardiovascular deaths). The occurrence of MACE in patients with vitamin C levels below 32 micromol/l and between 32 and 60 micromol/l was 3.9 times greater and 3.03 times greater, respectively, compared to those with levels above 60 micromol/l. Therefore, the authors of this publication suggested that low vitamin C levels predict adverse cardiovascular outcomes among maintenance hemodialysis patients.

Myint, Phyo Kyaw et al. **"Plasma vitamin C concentrations predict risk of incident stroke over 10 y in 20 649 participants of the European Prospective Investigation into Cancer Norfolk prospective population study."** The American journal of clinical nutrition 87 1 (2008): 64-9 .

The authors of this publication examined the relation between baseline plasma vitamin C concentrations and risk of incident stroke in a British population. This population-based prospective study included over 20,000 men and women aged 40-79 years without prevalent stroke. These participants were followed for 10 years. There were 448 strokes during this time. As it turned out, plasma vitamin C concentrations in the top quartile were linked to a 42% lower risk of stroke compared to the values in the lowest quartile. This result was independent from age, sex, smoking, body mass index, systolic blood pressure, physical activity, prevent diabetes, etc.

Other analyzes also suggested that the risk of stroke decreased by 19% when comparing those with the highest and lowest vitamin C intakes, and that for the difference between the highest and lowest circulating vitamin C concentration, the risk was 38% lower.

The onset of atherosclerosis

To begin with, local vitamin C deficiencies in the arterial walls can lead to membrane degeneration.

Gore, Ira et al. "**Endothelial changes produced by ascorbic acid deficiency in guinea pigs.**" Archives of pathology 80 4 (1965): 371-6 .

In this study, scientists induced scurvy in guinea pigs by giving them food lacking vitamin C. Using an electron microscope, they found that in these guinea pigs a lack of vitamin C led to a separation of endothelial cells, depletion of subendothelial collagen and reduction of cytoplasmic organelles.

What happened to these guinea pigs is a good start for atherosclerosis. When the cells that line the inner walls of a blood vessel begin to break down, these tissues thicken. And this is when dissolved substances (such as cholesterol or calcium) begin to accumulate. This influence of vitamin C on vascular endothelial functions should be kept in mind. Importantly, such an influence was also confirmed by many other newer studies. For example, studies have shown that ascorbic acid also potentiates nitric oxide (NO) synthesis in cultured human endothelial cells. This can protect the vessels against altered vasoconstriction and coagulation abnormalities.

Now we will look at risk factors for coronary heart disease and their relationship to vitamin C. The most popular risk factors for coronary artery disease include: age, gender, high blood pressure, high cholesterol (also the level of LDL to HDL), smoking, diabetes, triglycerides, homocysteine, high-sensitivity C-reactive protein (hs-CRP) and physical activity.

Cholesterol

In the past, a link between cholesterol and atherosclerosis has been established and LDL has come to be seen as the causative factor. The exact mechanism, however, was unknown. The theory that atherosclerosis is mainly caused by fat was developed largely through epidemiological studies. One of the most important contributors to this was Ancel Keys. In the 1950s, he collected data from six countries and drew a correlation between mortality from coronary heart disease (CHD) and fat consumption. A few years later, he created a new study called the "Seven Countries" study in which he assigned an atherogenic role only to saturated fat. The widespread lipid hypothesis proposed that hypercholesterolemia was a causative factor in human atherosclerosis. Over the past 50 years, there have also been studies suggesting that lowering cholesterol with drugs or diet reduces the risk of coronary heart disease and fatal heart attacks. On the other hand, there were more and more voices suggesting otherwise.

Ravnskov, Uffe et al. **"LDL-C does not cause cardiovascular disease: a comprehensive review of the current literature."** Expert Review of Clinical Pharmacology 11 (2018): 959 - 970.

In this comprehensive review of the current literature from 2018, researchers indicated that not only is high cholesterol not associated with a higher incidence of heart disease, but neither is LDL cholesterol. We can read that "The idea that high cholesterol levels in the blood are the main cause of CVD (cardiovascular disease) is impossible because people with low levels become just as atherosclerotic as people with high levels and their risk of suffering from CVD is the same or higher" and "Despite the fact that LDL-C is routinely referred to as the 'bad cholesterol', we have shown that high LDL-C levels appear to be unrelated to the risk of CVD, both in FH (familial hypercholesterolemia) individuals and in the general population and that the benefit from the use of cholesterol-lowering drugs is questionable."

Thus, despite these convincing premises, which are becoming more and more visible (but still rare in the medical community) and trustworthy, we will look at several studies on vitamin C and this topic.

Gc, Willis. **"An experimental study of intimal ground substance in atherosclerosis."** Canadian Medical Association Journal 69 (1953): 17-22.

Dr. G. Christopher Willis, in a study on guinea pigs, concluded that ascorbic acid deficiency in these animals can lead to atherosclerosis with normal cholesterol levels (= be the only cause of the disease). He also added that this form of atherosclerosis closely resembles that found in humans. Intraperitoneal vitamin C, in turn, greatly inhibits atherosclerosis of cholesterol feeding in guinea pigs.

In another study also in guinea pigs, Emil Ginter achieved a similar result in the form of atherosclerosis with vitamin C deficiency. Importantly, cholesterol and triglycerides were present in the animals' aortas despite not adding cholesterol to the food.

Maeda, Nobuyo et al. **"Aortic wall damage in mice unable to synthesize ascorbic acid."** Proceedings of the National Academy of Sciences of the United States of America 97 2 (2000): 841-6 .

In mice, the authors inactivated an essential gene for the enzyme necessary to synthesize vitamin C. So these animals became, like humans, dependent on dietary vitamin C. When plasma ascorbic acid decreased, there were significant increases in total cholesterol and decreases in high density lipoprotein cholesterol (HDL). They also found that "the most striking effects of the marginal dietary vitamin C were alterations in the wall of aorta, evidenced by the disruption of elastic laminae, smooth muscle cell proliferation, and focal endothelial desquamation of the luminal surface."

Ginter E, Cerná O, Budlovský J, Baláz V, Hrubá F, Roch V, Sasko E. **Effect of ascorbic acid on plasma cholesterol in humans in a long-term experiment.** Int J Vitam Nutr Res. 1977;47(2):123-34. PMID: 881295.

This study enrolled 82 men and women aged 50-75 years who received 1 gram of vitamin C (2x500 mg) per day. Cholesterol levels were tested at the beginning of the study and after 3 months. As it turned out; the higher the initial cholesterolemia, the greater the hypocholesterolemic effect of ascorbic acid. People whose initial cholesterol level was above 230 mg% continued the study for another 9 months. Ascorbic acid was found to further significantly depress cholesterolemia. The greatest decrease in cholesterol level was noted in patients with hypertension and a mean starting cholesterolemia value of 272 mg%. After a year of vitamin C supplementation, this level dropped to an average of 218 mg%. Overall, a year-long administration of ascorbic acid produced a remarkable and clinically notable decline in cholesterolemia in over 60% of the participants.

McRae, M.P. (2008). **Vitamin C supplementation lowers serum low-density lipoprotein cholesterol and triglycerides: a meta-analysis of 13 randomized controlled trials.** Journal of chiropractic medicine, 7 2, 48-58 .

The purpose of this meta-analysis of randomized controlled trials was to investigate the effect of vitamin C supplementation on LDL and HDL cholesterol as well as triglycerides. The study included 13 trials in which people with hypercholesterolaemia received vitamin C in an amount of at least 500 mg/day for between 3 and 24 weeks. The pooled estimate of effect for ascorbic acid supplementation for LDL was -7.9 mg/dL. For HDL, it was statistically insignificant 1.1 mg/ml. In the case of triglycerides, the pooled estimate of effect for vitamin C was -20.1 mg/dL. In summary, vitamin C in an amount of at least 500 mg/day for a minimum of 4 weeks significantly reduced LDL and triglycerides. However, it had no significant effect on HDL.

Summarizing the above, I will come back to what I mentioned at the beginning of the chapter. We have solid evidence to suggest that cholesterol build-up in the membranes occurs in areas with a local vitamin C deficiency. In other words, this detrimental process is initiated by scurvy of blood vessel tissues (e.g. of arterial wall). This is when degeneration occurs. I wrote "local" because vitamin C deficiency does not have to affect the whole body in this case.

Triglycerides

NHANES 1999-2008 showed that overall prevalence of hypertriglyceridemia in the adult population in the United States is about 31%. Furthermore, the prevalence of triglyceride levels above 150 mg/dL is almost twice as high in people with metabolic syndrome. Since a meta-analysis previously showed that vitamin C is capable of lowering triglyceride levels, we now look at this type of lipid a little. Triglycerides are strongly associated with cardiovascular diseases, such as coronary artery disease and atherosclerosis.

Miller, Michael et al. "**Impact of triglyceride levels beyond low-density lipoprotein cholesterol after acute coronary syndrome in the PROVE IT-TIMI 22 trial.**" Journal of the American College of Cardiology 51 7 (2008): 724-30 .

A post hoc analysis performed by the PROVE-IT TIMI 22 showed an association between hypertriglyceridemia and acute cardiovascular (CV) events. The study itself involved 4,162 patients hospitalized for acute coronary syndrome (ACS) and randomized to atorvastatin 80 mg or pravastatin 40 mg daily (both of these drugs are statins working by slowing the production of cholesterol in the body). Various associations between triglycerides and LDL and the composite end point of death, myocardial infarction, and recurrent ACS were assessed after 30 days of intervention. It turned out that even when patients who had sustained an acute myocardial infarction and achieved LDL level below 70 mg/dl with a statin, a triglycerides level greater than 200 mg/dl was associated with a 40% greater risk of an acute cardiovascular event compared with those participants with a triglycerides level below 200 mg/dl.

Additionally, other studies have shown that even with lower triglyceride levels (100-200 mg/dl) there is a linear rise in risk of cardiovascular events as triglycerides increase.

Now we turn to publications showing the effect of vitamin C on triglyceride levels. Before doing so, I will briefly explain one thing that will appear in the next study. Lipoprotein lipase (LPL) is an extracellular enzyme that degrades circulating triglycerides in the bloodstream. A decrease in LPL activity is associated with an increase in plasma triglycerides and decrease in HDL cholesterol. This, as we can already guess, is disadvantageous.

Sokoloff, Boris et al. **"AGING, ATHEROSCLEROSIS AND ASCORBIC ACID METABOLISM *."** Journal of the American Geriatrics Society 14 (1966): n. pag.

In this study, scientists examined the effects of ascorbic acid on blood lipids in rabbits, rats and man. The rabbits were divided into three groups: the control group, the one that received 100 mg of cholesterol per kg of body weight, and the one that received cholesterol plus 150 mg of ascorbic acid per kg of body weight. After 8 months the mean total plasma cholesterol was 88.5 mg %, 1234mg% and 308 mg%, respectively. As for the triglycerides, they were 26 mg%, 195 mg% and 89 mg%, respectively. In the second group examination showed pronounced atheroma-like lesions in the vascular system. In turn, in the group where ascorbic acid was administered, they were only slight. The results for the rats were similar. In the case of people, 234 subjects were given 1.5 to 3 grams of ascorbic acid for 4 to 30 months. In a group of 60 patients with hypercholesterolaemia, the supplementation of ascorbic acid resulted in marked improvement in 50 participants. More specifically; lipoprotein lipase (LPL) activity increased by 100% and triglycerides declined by 50% to 70%.

Erden, F et al. **"Ascorbic acid effect on some lipid fractions in human beings."** Acta vitaminologica et enzymologica 7 1-2 (1985): 131-7.

In this study, scientists administered to 50 subjects 2 grams of vitamin C per day at regular time intervals for 2 months. Blood samples were collected at the beginning and end of the intervention. During this time, there was a significant decrease in cholesterol levels. Similarly with triglycerides, the level of these lipids also decreased. On the other hand, there has been a significant increase in HDL cholesterol levels.

I would also like to add that in studies on guinea pigs, the administration of an adequate amount of vitamin C also leads to a reduction in triglycerides. In humans, in turn, plasma vitamin C levels and triglyceride levels appear to be inversely correlated. In other words, the more vitamin C, the lower the triglyceride concentration.

Homocysteine

Another risk factor for atherosclerosis that we will consider is homocysteine. An increased homocysteine level promotes atherosclerosis. Levels of this type of amino acid are commonly significantly higher in people with coronary artery disease than in those without this disease. One of the many causes of high homocysteine levels (such as vitamin B12, B9, and B6 deficiencies, which I discussed in more detail in my previous book) is possibly vitamin C deficiency.

Nappo, Francesco et al. **"Impairment of endothelial functions by acute hyperhomocysteinemia and reversal by antioxidant vitamins."** JAMA 281 22 (1999): 2113-8 .

In this study, scientists evaluated the effect of acute hyperhomocysteinemia with and without antioxidant vitamin pretreatment on cardiovascular risk factors. Three groups were created. The first group got oral methionine (homocysteine is made from the breakdown of methionine) with fruit juice, the second group got methionine with juice and antioxidant vitamins (800 IU of vitamin E and 1000 mg of vitamin C) and the third got only fruit juice (placebo). The oral methionine load increased the mean homocysteine level from 10.5 μmol/L at baseline to 27.1 μmol/L at 4 hours. Supplementation with methionine alone resulted in coagulation and alteration of the adhesive properties of endothelium. As it turned out, no such effect was observed when vitamins with antioxidant properties were also administered. It simply means that these vitamins prevented the effects of hyperhomocysteinemia.

Chambers, J C et al. **"Demonstration of rapid onset vascular endothelial dysfunction after hyperhomocysteinemia: an effect reversible with vitamin C therapy."** Circulation 99 9 (1999): 1156-60 .

A similar study investigated the effect of pretreatment with vitamin C when patients had their homocysteine levels elevated. Higher levels were achieved with methionine supplementation (L-methionine 100 mg/kg). There was also a group that, apart from methionine, received 1 gram of vitamin C. Pretreatment with vitamin C had a positive effect on flow-mediated dilatation. Vitamin C contributed to the fact that the blood flowed freely, the arteries remained permeable, and the muscles in the arteries did not contract excessively. Adding the words of the authors themselves: "We conclude that an elevation in homocysteine concentration is associated with an acute impairment of vascular endothelial function that can be prevented by pretreatment with vitamin C in healthy subjects. Our results support the hypothesis that the adverse effects of homocysteine on vascular endothelial cells are mediated through oxidative stress mechanisms."

Histamine

Another risk factor for atherosclerosis that is worth paying attention to is histamine. Although this is not a factor that is often taken into account. Histamine is an organic nitrogenous compound taking part, among others, in inflammation and allergic reactions, is a neurotransmitter and stimulates the secretion of gastric acid. This compound has also been linked to atherosclerosis.

Majno, G., & Palade, G.E. (1961). **STUDIES ON INFLAMMATION: I. The Effect of Histamine and Serotonin on Vascular Permeability:** An Electron Microscopic Study. Journal of Cell Biology, 11, 571-605.

In this study, administration of histamine resulted in numerous endothelial openings present in blood vessels in rats. Interestingly, a similar phenomenon was mentioned by me at the very beginning of this chapter, where vitamin C deficiency contributed to the separation of endothelial cells in guinea pigs. In the above study in rats, it was also found that these endothelial openings can leak and pass plasma.

Other studies in mice have shown that histamine is involved in the development of atherosclerosis by regulating gene expression of inflammatory modulators. As it turns out, histamine participates not only in acute inflammatory responses but also in chronic inflammation specific to atherosclerosis. Moreover, studies in rabbits have shown that the administration of chlorpheniramine (an antihistamine substance) slows down the growth of atherosclerosis in these animals. Also vitamin C is able to normalize the elevated level of histamine as it is essential for the metabolic breakdown of this compound.

Clemetson CA. **Histamine and ascorbic acid in human blood.** J Nutr. 1980 Apr;110(4):662-8. doi: 10.1093/jn/110.4.662. PMID: 7365537.

In this study, supplementation with 1 gram of ascorbic acid for three days resulted in a reduction of the blood histamine level in every subject. Analysis of 437 human blood samples showed that when plasma vitamin C levels fall below 1 mg/100 ml, histamine levels increase exponentially as the ascorbic acid level decreases. Furthermore, when the level of this vitamin drops below 0.7 mg/100 ml, there is a highly significant increase in histamine.

Johnston, Carol S. et al. "**Vitamin C depletion is associated with alterations in blood histamine and plasma free carnitine in adults.**" Journal of the American College of Nutrition 15 6 (1996): 586-91.

In the above study, scientists investigated the effects of vitamin C in low doses and doses above the recommended dietary allowance on histamine and carnitine levels. Two groups with low levels of vitamin C (but without scurvy) were on diets low in this vitamin for three weeks. After this time, vitamin C supplementation was gradually (weekly) increased (and measurements were made). The first group was getting 10, 30 and 60 mg of vitamin C per day, while the second group was getting 10, 125 and 250 mg for weeks 1, 2 and 3, respectively. In the first group, vitamin C supplementation had no effect on histamine levels. In the second group, on the other hand, the histamine levels were inversely related to vitamin C status. Therefore, the authors concluded: "Thus utilizing scurvy as an end-point to determine vitamin C requirements may not provide adequate vitamin C to promote optimal health and well-being." At this point, I must point out that the recommended doses of vitamin C are just those that are mainly intended to prevent scurvy and not to provide sufficiency for the entire body. This study is only one of many examples of the truth of this statement.

Clemetson, C. Alan B.. "**The key role of histamine in the development of atherosclerosis and coronary heart disease**." Medical hypotheses 52 1 (1999): 1-8 .

Dr. Clemetson claimed in general that histamine plays a key role in the development of atherosclerosis. He indicated that a high level of histamine causes separation of vascular endothelial cells. And this is just histaminemia and ascorbate depletion together cause damage to the arterial endothelium and predispose to atherosclerosis.

Lipoprotein(a)

Another important risk factor for atherosclerosis is lipoprotein(a). This lipoprotein was discovered in 1963 and was slightly disregarded until it was found to be associated with heart health. Lipoprotein(a) has repair and strengthening properties (although when there is not too much of it, more on that later) similar to vitamin C. For this reason, Dr. Matthias Rath and Linus Pauling believed that this substance plays the role of vitamin C. They also found that animals that do not synthesize vitamin C have the highest levels of this lipoprotein and on the other hand animals that are able to produce sufficient amounts of vitamin C do not need Lp(a) in any significant amount. The researchers presented a new concept according to which, due to endothelial degeneration (because of vitamin C deficiency), there is a deposition of Lp(a) in the arterial wall to compensate for its structural weakness. Overcompensation (i.e., deposition) of lipoproteins(a) on the walls of the arteries, however, lead to atherosclerosis. It is also worth noting that along with Lp(a) there appears also fibrinogen (which supports clotting), further converted to fibrin (which is part of the clot).

von Eckardstein, Arnold et al. "**Lipoprotein(a) further increases the risk of coronary events in men with high global cardiovascular risk**." Journal of the American College of Cardiology 37 2 (2001): 434-9 .

In this prospective population study, scientists wanted to assess the role of higher levels of lipoprotein(a) as a coronary risk factor.

788 male participants aged 35 to 65 years were followed for 10 years. During this time, 44 people suffered myocardial infarction. Other traditional cardiovascular risk factors were also taken into account, and people with lipoprotein(a) levels above 0.2 g/l (20 mg/dl) were found to have 2.7 times greater risk of a coronary event than those with levels below 0.2g/l. Additionally, for example, in men with hypertension, this risk was further increased.

In a few studies, the relationship between lipoprotein(a) and the risk of atherosclerosis has been examined causal and independent. Furthermore, there have also been several studies showing a causal link between Lp(a) and, for example, calcific aortic valve stenosis.

Cha, John et al. **"Hypoascorbemia induces atherosclerosis and vascular deposition of lipoprotein(a) in transgenic mice."** American journal of cardiovascular disease 5 1 (2015): 53-62 .

This study was conducted in transgenic mice that could not synthesize vitamin C. These mice were divided into three groups; completely deprived of vitamin C, receiving low and receiving high doses of vitamin C daily. When the mice experienced hypoascorbemia and scurvy, lipoprotein(a) accumulated in the vascular walls. It was then that atherosclerosis developed. It should also be noted that the animals were not on any high-lipid diets. The degree of lesions was found to be inversely related to the intake of vitamin C. Therefore, in mice that received the highest amounts of vitamin C, the least Lp(a) was deposited. Cha, Niedzwiecki and Rath concluded: "These data indicate that the structural impairment of the vascular wall in hypoascorbemia and scurvy by itself is sufficient for the deposition of Lp (a) and the development of atherosclerosis."

Pauling L. **Third case report on lysine-ascorbate amelioration of angina pectoris.** J Orthomolecular Med 1993;8:137-138.

Linus Pauling also suggested that lysine may increase the effectiveness of vitamin C treatment. This essential amino acid can bind circulating Lp(a) and thus prevent these lipoproteins from binding to the arterial walls. The publication above presents one of three cases of effective angina (usually caused by coronary heart disease) control with vitamin C and lysine. Such results were obtained thanks to supplementation with vitamin C and lysine in doses of 3-6 grams a day, and the response to treatment appeared within two to four weeks. Apart from this publication, Dr. Rath also proposed adding proline for a more effective treatment.

Earlier I also mentioned fibrogen which many studies show is strongly associated with coronary artery disease. This protein plays a significant role in blood clotting and affects its viscosity. Excess is especially dangerous. Few studies have found that vitamin C and fibrinogen levels are inversely proportional.

Bordia, A K et al. **"Acute effect of ascorbic acid on fibrinolytic activity."** Atherosclerosis 30 4 (1978): 351-4 .

In this study, scientists investigated the effect of vitamin C on fibrinolytic activity (which prevents blood clots from growing further). All forty men were getting 1 gram of vitamin C per day. In healthy men, serum vitamin C levels increased by about 71%, while the fibrinolytic activity increased to 137% at 6 h. A similar increase in fibrinolytic activity was observed in participants with coronary artery disease. In the third group, when in addition to vitamin C, also 100 grams of fat were given fibrinolytic activity increased by 64% above the fasting level. This suggests that vitamin C prevented the decline in this activity.

Hypertension

Hypertension is a well-known factor in the development of atherosclerosis. Almost half (47%) of American adults have this condition. High blood pressure can enhance atherosclerotic processes in such a way that it overloads the abnormal structure of the blood vessel walls (lacking collagen), leading to further degeneration and, consequently, to atherosclerosis. As I mentioned at the very beginning, it is very likely that vitamin C is responsible for this inadequate structure. When there is a lack of vitamin C, properly formed collagen begins to break down in blood vessels. Wound healing is not happening properly. Scars also require adequate amounts of vitamin C to form correctly.

However, vitamin C may also be crucial in this aspect for another reason. As it turns out, vitamin C (among many other substances, such as, for example, potassium and magnesium) can lower blood pressure.

Oregon State University. **"Vitamin C Can Reduce High Blood Pressure, Study Finds**." ScienceDaily. ScienceDaily, 21 December 1999. <www.sciencedaily.com/releases/1999/12/991221080724.htm>.

Scientists at the Boston University School of Medicine and the Linus Pauling Institute at Oregon State University wanted to study the effects of vitamin C on blood pressure. For this placebo-controlled, double-blind study, they included 45 participants with high blood pressure (diastolic blood pressure over 90 and systolic blood pressure over 140 mm Hg). Patients took 500 mg of vitamin C. After the first month of supplementation, it turned out that the systolic, diastolic and mean blood pressures all decreased by about 9%. In other words, the mean systolic pressure dropped from 155 to 142, diastolic from 87 to 79 and blood pressure from 110 to 100 mm Hg. Furthermore, the authors added that the blood pressure lowering effect of vitamin C only seems to affect people with blood pressure higher than recommended.

Juraschek, Stephen P. et al. **"Effects of vitamin C supplementation on blood pressure: a meta-analysis of randomized controlled trials**." The American journal of clinical nutrition 95 5 (2012): 1079-88 .

For this meta-analysis, scientists analyzed twenty-nine randomized controlled trials that looked at the effects of vitamin C on blood pressure. The median dose was 500 mg of vitamin C per day and the median duration of the studies was 8 weeks. The pooled change in systolic blood pressure (SBP) was -3.84 mm Hg and in diastolic blood pressure (DBP) was -1.48 mm Hg. In the case of participants with hypertension, SBP was -4.85 mm Hg and DBP -1.67 mm Hg. Thus as the study showd vitamin C is able to lower blood pressure in the short term. Long-term studies of the effects of vitamin C on this risk factor are lacking.

In addition, other studies in a large group of people found that the probability of having high blood pressure was even 22% lower for subjects in the top quartiles of plasma vitamin C levels compared to the bottom quartiles.

Infections

Another factor that may contribute to atherosclerosis is inflammation caused by infections. These infections can, of course, come from different origins. One of them, well known and documented, is periodontal disease. When this disease is left untreated, various microbes enter the bloodstream and attack the walls of the arteries. If our immunity is weak (we have vitamin C deficiency, for example, among other things), this may have serious health consequences in the future.

Morrison, Howard I. et al. "**Periodontal Disease and Risk of Fatal Coronary Heart and Cerebrovascular Diseases.**" European Journal of Preventive Cardiology 6 (1999): 11 - 7.

In this retrospective cohort study scientists examined the relationship between periodontal disease and the risk for coronary heart disease (CHD). 10,368 participants without self-reported coronary heart disease (CHD) and 11,251 participants without cerebrovascular (CVD) disease aged 35-84 years were followed. Finally, 416 deaths from CHD and 182 deaths from CVD were included in the analysis. After adjusting for other risk factors, it turned out that there is a statistically significant association between periodontal disease and risk of fatal CHD. People with severe gingivitis were 2.15 times more likely to die from CHD and those with edentulous status 1.9 times more.

Other prospective studies also suggested a 1.5 to 2.5 fold increased risk of developing complications of atherosclerosis when patients had periodontal disease at baseline. Interestingly, at the beginning of the 21st century, the DNA of some microbes characteristic of periodontal disease was also discovered on atherosclerotic plaques.

Wiesel, J. (1906). **Die Erkrankungen arterieller Gefäße im Verlaufe akuter Infektionen.** Z Heilkd, 27, 262-294.

Researchers more than 100 years ago, after performing

an autopsy, found that various microbial agents can cause substantial damage to the vascular walls.

Publications, in turn, from this century suggested that the endothelium is significantly exposed in the case of infection. Infections affecting blood vessels can be caused by bacteria such as H. pylori or C. pneumoniae and viruses such as cytomegalovirus, Coxsackie B virus, enteroviruses, H. simplex, hepatitis A or Epstein-Barr virus. For example, scientists found DNA of herpes simplex virus in the coronary arteries in 38% of people who died from myocardial infarction. Infection of endothelial cells may lead to acute complications such as thrombosis and hemorrhage, when chronic it may also result in atherosclerosis or vasculitis (inflammation of the blood vessels).

Also, high levels of C-reactive protein (CRP) are often associated with atherosclerosis, which can also result from infections. However, there is no certainty about the causality itself in this aspect. Scientists mention several roles of CRP in this process, such as for example; promoting the development of atherosclerotic lesions, leading to endothelial cell dysfunction (by disrupting endothelial nitric oxide synthase activity) or disrupting the endothelial vascular activity. Additionally, CRP has also been detected in atherosclerotic plaques. Vitamin C can significantly reduce the level of this protein.

Block, Gladys et al. **"Vitamin C treatment reduces elevated C-reactive protein."** Free radical biology & medicine 46 1 (2009): 70-7 .

In this study, scientists wanted to find out if vitamin C and vitamin E were able to lower the level of C-reactive protein (CRP). For this purpose, 396 healthy nonsmokers were randomized to three groups. One group got 1000 mg of vitamin C per day, the second group got 800 IU of vitamin E, and the third group got a placebo, for two months. Due to the fact that the median CRP level was low (0.85 mg/L), the effect of the treatment was insignificant after taking into account all participants. However, it was different when different baseline CRP levels were included. When including those participants who have an increased risk of cardiovascular disease or CRP greater than or equal to 1.0 mg/L, vitamin C reduced the median CRP by 25.3% compared to the placebo group. As the authors added, these effects were similar to those of statins. It is also disquieting that among the obese, 75% had CRP greater than or equal to 1.0 mg/l.

After the chapter on vitamin C and the infections, I do not need to repeat the importance of this vitamin in our immunity. The body then needs much more vitamin C and the resources shrink quickly. It will come as no surprise that vitamin C can reduce the risk of atherosclerosis also in this regard.

There are also other risk factors for atherosclerosis, such as for example diabetes or smoking. Later in the book we will also look at them in more detail.

Varbo, Anette et al. "**Extreme nonfasting remnant cholesterol vs extreme LDL cholesterol as contributors to cardiovascular disease and all-cause mortality in 90000 individuals from the general population.**" Clinical chemistry 61 3 (2015): 533-43 .

Wakabayashi, I., & Daimon, T. (2019). **Comparison of discrimination for cardio-metabolic risk by different cut-off values of the ratio of triglycerides to HDL cholesterol.** Lipids in Health and Disease, 18.

As evidenced partially by the previous studies I've presented on vitamin C, it is also likely to lower lesser-known (but probably the best) predictors for cardiovascular disease like remnant cholesterol and the triglyceride/HDL cholesterol ratio (TG/HDL-C ratio).

CHAPTER 49:
RHEUMATOID
ARTHRITIS

In the section on vitamin D, I wrote that in the case of rheumatoid arthritis (RA), this vitamin can be very effective in both prevention and treatment. The situation seems to be similar with vitamin C. This is due to the various properties of this vitamin. Vitamin C reduces inflammation (lower levels of inflammatory cytokines), closely related to rheumatoid arthritis. Vitamin C modulates the autoimmune response because, as we know, RA is an autoimmune disease. Moreover, vitamin C can protect cartilage as it is essential for collagen synthesis. Studies have shown that the best therapeutic results can be obtained with vitamin C given intravenously.

Mikirova, Nina A. et al. **"Effect of high dose intravenous ascorbic acid on the level of inflammation in patients with rheumatoid arthritis.**" (2012).

In this study, which was conducted at the Riordan Clinic, scientists investigated the effects of intravenous vitamin C on patients with rheumatoid arthritis. Eleven patients characterized by moderate to high levels of the inflammation marker CRP were given intravenous vitamin C in the amount of 7.5, 15 or 25 grams. Before treatment, the mean CRP level was 9.4 mg/l, while after treatment, the mean CRP level was 6.4 mg/l (decrease by 32%). Moreover, for the nine people who responded best to IV vitamin C, the mean decrease in CRP was 44%. For example, in the sixth patient, the CRP level dropped steadily from 12.6 mg/L to 1.4 mg/L. This person had twenty vitamin C infusions of 15 grams over a 130 day period.

Carr, Anitra C. et al. **"Parenteral vitamin C relieves chronic**

fatigue and pain in a patient with rheumatoid arthritis and mononeuritis multiplex secondary to CNS vasculitis." Case Reports in Clinical Pathology 2 (2015): 57.

It is also worth mentioning the case report of other scientists. They wanted to investigate the effect of intravenous vitamin C on chronic fatigue and pain in a patient with multiple morbidities. The patient was a 47-year-old female with rheumatoid arthritis and mononeuritis multiplex, secondary to central nervous system vasculitis. The woman had symptoms such as chronic fatigue, pain and insomnia. She was given 50 grams of intravenous vitamin C followed by two more infusions about one week apart. The quality of life questionnaire indicated a significant improvement in the patient's health, especially in terms of physical functioning and cognitive functions. In addition, there was a significant decrease in symptoms such as pain, insomnia and fatigue. No adverse effects of the intravenous administration of vitamin C were observed.

CHAPTER 50: PAIN

As was seen in a previous study, vitamin C can reduce pain in rheumatoid arthritis. However, scientists have found that vitamin C has this effect in many other diseases as well. For example, in Paget's disease, a chronic bone disease involving the development of abnormalities in the mechanism of bone formation and breakdown (resorption), or a complex regional pain syndrome.

Basu TK, Smethurst M, Gillett MB, Donaldson D, Jordan SJ, Williams DC, Hicklin JA. **Ascorbic acid therapy for the relief of bone pain in Paget's disease.** Acta Vitaminol Enzymol. 1978;32(1-4):45-9. PMID: 582875.

In this study, Basu, et al, investigated the effects of oral doses of vitamin C on Paget's disease. Sixteen patients with painful Paget's disease of the bone were enrolled in the study. The daily dose of oral vitamin C was 3 grams. 50% of patients experienced a decrease in pain within a period of 5 to 7 days after starting this vitamin therapy. Additionally, a daily dose of 3 grams of vitamin C resulted in a complete elimination of pain in 20% of the patients. The results therefore indicated the potential efficacy of vitamin C in gram doses in at least alleviating the symptoms of this disease.

Besse JL, Gadeyne S, Galand-Desmé S, Lerat JL, Moyen B. **Effect of vitamin C on prevention of complex regional pain syndrome type I in foot and ankle surgery.** Foot Ankle Surg 2009;15:179-82.

Complex regional pain syndrome (CRPS) is a form of chronic pain that usually occurs after surgery or injury, and affects the leg or arm. The authors of the above publication wanted to assess whether vitamin C can prevent CRPS I in foot and ankle surgery. 392 patients (and 420 feet) were enrolled in the study; 185 was in Group 1 and 235 in Group 2. Contrary to group 1, group 2 was given preventive vitamin C in the amount of 1 gram a day. As it turned out, CRPS I occurred in 9.6% of participants in group 1 and in only 1.7% of participants in group 2. The results of this study showed the high effectiveness of vitamin C in preventing CRPS I of the foot and ankle.

CHAPTER 51:
DIABETES

Vitamin C plays an important role in diabetes and deficiencies of this vitamin are common in this disease. First, I must mention that vitamin C competes with glucose for entering the cell. This means that the more glucose we have, the less vitamin C. On the other hand, people with diabetes often have a problem with controlling glucose. This fact and the occurring hyperglycemia can lead to a vitamin C deficiency. Second, diabetic patients may also have low insulin levels. Insulin, in turn, promotes cellular uptake of vitamin C. Eventually, studies have shown that supplementation with this essential substance can be of great help in controlling and treating this condition.

D, P., Puvvada, R.C., & M, V.A. (2020). **Association of vitamin C status in diabetes mellitus: prevalence and predictors of vitamin C deficiency**. Future Journal of Pharmaceutical Sciences, 6.

The authors of this prospective cross-sectional study aimed to assess the prevalence of vitamin C deficiency in diabetes patients. For this reason, 292 participants were examined and categorized into three groups according to their vitamin C levels. Finally, the scientists came to some important conclusions. Vitamin C deficiency concerned over 55.1% of diabetic patients. An inverse relationship has been found between vitamin C levels and fasting blood sugar levels. In addition, those with inadequate and deficient vitamin C levels had a significant increase in the systolic blood pressure levels. Total cholesterol was also inversely related to vitamin C levels.

Afkhami-Ardekani M, Shojaoddiny-Ardekani A. **Effect of**

vitamin C on blood glucose, serum lipids & serum insulin in type 2 diabetes patients. Indian J Med Res. 2007 Nov;126(5):471-4. PMID: 18160753.

In an earlier study, scientists found an inverse correlation between fasting blood sugar levels and vitamin C levels. In this study, in turn, scientists examined the effects of different doses of vitamin C on blood glucose and serum lipids. 84 patients with type 2 diabetes have been divided into two groups. One group was given 500 mg per day and the other group 1000 mg for six weeks. As it turned out, vitamin C administered at 1 gram per day caused a significant decrease in fasting blood sugar, triglyceride, LDL and glycated hemoglobin. Importantly, such an effect was not observed with the administration of vitamin C in an amount of 500 mg per day.

Harding, Anne-Helen et al. **"Plasma vitamin C level, fruit and vegetable consumption, and the risk of new-onset type 2 diabetes mellitus: the European prospective investigation of cancer--Norfolk prospective study."** Archives of internal medicine 168 14 (2008): 1493-9.

Based on a population-based prospective cohort, researchers aimed to assess the relationship between fruit and vegetable intake, plasma vitamin C level and the risk of incident type 2 diabetes. The participants of this cohort were 21 831 healthy people aged 40 to 75 years with determined levels of vitamin C and the assessed consumption of vegetables and fruits. During 12 years of follow-up, 735 cases of diabetes occurred. Scientists noted a strong inverse association between plasma vitamin C level and diabetes risk. People with the highest levels of vitamin C had a reduced risk of diabetes by up to 38%. Fruit and vegetables were less associated with diabetes risk reduction, but still inversely.

Sarji, K. E. et al. **"Decreased platelet vitamin C in diabetes mellitus: possible role in hyperaggregation."** Thrombosis research 15 5-6 (1979): 639-50.

Increased platelet aggregation leads often to the angiopathy (damage to nerve fibers) that occurs in diabetics. These scientists investigated the effects of ascorbic acid both in vitro and in vivo on platelet aggregation. Overall, the vitamin C level was significantly lower in diabetics than in normals. Moreover, vitamin C levels in washed platelets from diabetics were also significantly lower than from normals. In turn, the addition of vitamin C resulted in an inhibition of platelet aggregation in vitro. In vivo, non-smoker men received 2 grams of vitamin C per day for seven days. These men experienced marked inhibition of aggregation.

Lazareth I, Hubert S, Michon-Pasturel U, Priollet P. **[Vitamin C deficiency and leg ulcers. A case control study]**. Journal des Maladies Vasculaires. 2007 Apr;32(2):96-99. DOI: 10.1016/j.jmv.2007.02.003. PMID: 17475430.

Up to 15% of people with diabetes develop a non healing skin wound on their legs defined as chronic leg ulcers. Therefore, French scientists decided to investigate whether vitamin C deficiency affects patients with this ailment. They took blood samples from 42 patients with chronic leg ulcers and 37 patients without chronic leg ulcers (but with peripheral vascular disease, or hypertension, or connective disorders). The mean level of vitamin C in people with chronic leg ulcers was 23.9 µmol/l, whereas in the control group it was 33.8 µmol/l. In the control group, however, smoking was more frequent. Hypovitaminosis C (6-26 µmol/l) in the leg ulcers group was present in 23.8% and 16.2% in the control group. Scurvy was found in 26.2% of people in the leg ulcers group versus 5.4% in the control group. Also, C reactive protein levels were higher in the leg ulcers group and were 31.8 mg versus 9.3 mg in the control group.

CHAPTER 52:
OBESITY

Vitamin C deficiency may contribute, to some extent, to the massive obesity epidemic worldwide. This element is necessary for the synthesis of carnitine which in turn is essential for the utilization of fatty acids as energy. For example, in mice on an obesity-promoting diet, administration of vitamin C reduced body weight and mesenteric fat mass. Human studies have also shown vitamin C's beneficial properties against fat gain.

Johnston, Carol S. et al. "**Marginal vitamin C status is associated with reduced fat oxidation during submaximal exercise in young adults**." Nutrition & Metabolism 3 (2006): 35 - 35.

The authors of this publication evaluated the effects of vitamin C on fat oxidation during submaximal exercise. The study included 15 participants with marginal vitamin C levels and 7 participants with adequate vitamin C levels. Fat energy expenditure was determined in subjects during a submaximal, 60-minute treadmill test. Fat utilization during exercise was 25% lower among participants with marginal vitamin C status compared to participants with adequate vitamin C status. Moreover, the same scientists also conducted an 8-week double-blind, placebo-controlled, depletion-repletion trial. After four weeks of vitamin C depletion, participants took either 500 milligrams of vitamin C or a placebo daily for four weeks. After this time, the mean level of vitamin C in the supplementation group was 42 µmol/l, whereas in the placebo group the level was 10 µmol/l. In the case of the group that supplemented vitamin C, fatty acid utilization was 4-fold higher compared to the vitamin C depleted group.

CHAPTER 53: ALZHEIMER'S AND PARKINSON'S

One of the main factors accelerating the development of neurodegenerative diseases (such as Alzheimer's disease) is oxidative stress, i.e. imbalance between antioxidants and oxidants in favor of oxidants. Free radicals can alter the structure and function of lipids, proteins, and nucleic acids. Thus, they can also negatively affect many tissues and organs. The brain may be one of them given its vulnerable composition of easily oxidizable lipids. Vitamin C is obviously a potent antioxidant and can counteract it.

Engelhart, Marianne J. et al. **"Dietary intake of antioxidants and risk of Alzheimer disease."** JAMA 287 24 (2002): 3223-9 .

In this study, researchers investigated the relationship between antioxidant consumption and the risk of Alzheimer disease. Therefore, 5395 participants with an average age of at least 55 years and dementia-free at baseline were followed for 6 years. During this time, 197 people developed dementia, of whom 146 had Alzheimer disease. After many adjustments (including age, sex, alcohol intake, smoking habits etc.), researchers found that higher vitamin C intake is associated with a lower risk of Alzheimer disease. Participants with the highest levels of this vitamin had an 18% risk reduction.

Li, Yonghua et al. **"Effects of vitamins E and C combined with β-carotene on cognitive function in the elderly."** Experimental and Therapeutic Medicine 9 (2015): 1489 - 1493.

The authors of this publication aimed to investigate the effect of supplementation with vitamin C, E, combined with β-carotene on cognitive function in the elderly. The 276 people who completed the study were previously divided into five groups. Groups A, B, C, D were given 300 mg/day of vitamin C and 200 mg/day of vitamin E plus 16.7, 8.4, 5.6 or 0 mg/day of β-carotene, respectively. Group E, as a control group, received 5 mg/day of vitamin E. The study lasted 16 weeks. After this time, the researchers found that the Mini-Mental State Examination (MMSE) scores in groups A and B were significantly higher compared with the score in group E. The mean scores of Hasegawa Dementia Scale (HDS) tests in groups A and B also increased significantly compared to the results at the beginning of the study. Moreover, HDS scores in groups A and B were also significantly higher than in group E after treatment. Levels of amyloid-β (Aβ) peptides were lowered after treatment compared to levels before treatment (levels of Aβ peptides are usually elevated in Alzheimer's disease). In addition, plasma estradiol levels in group A after treatment were higher than before treatment and than in group E (the decline in estradiol is related to cognitive dysfunction and dementia).

Hantikainen, Essi et al. **"Dietary Antioxidants and the Risk of Parkinson Disease."** Neurology 96 (2021): e895 - e903.

These scientists investigated the relationship between baseline dietary antioxidants and risk of Parkinson disease in men and women. They followed nearly 44,000 people aged 18-94 from the large Swedish National March Cohort. Data on the amount of intake of vitamins C and E among others were collected at baseline. The mean follow-up was 17.6 years. During this time, 465 incidence cases of Parkinson disease were detected. The authors of this publication found that study participants who consumed the most vitamin C had a 32% decreased risk of Parkinson disease compared to those with the lowest intake. Moreover, the same reduced risk occurred in those who consumed the most vitamin E.

Quiroga, M Jabid et al. **"Ascorbate- and Zinc-Responsive Parkinsonism."** Annals of Pharmacotherapy 48 (2014): 1515 - 1520.

Among the few studies on the effects of vitamin C on Parkinson's disease, we have several case reports. This is one of them. This is a report of a 66-year-old man with Parkinson's disease, pleural effusion and bipolar disorder who was diagnosed with low levels of vitamin C and zinc. The man received both vitamin C and zinc intravenously, which led to a resolution of the movement disorder in less than 24 hours.

CHAPTER 54: DEPRESSION

Vitamin C deficiencies may promote depression as well as contribute to adverse mood and cognitive effects. There are at least a few reasons why this might be so. Vitamin C plays an important role in modulating the synthesis of neurotransmitters and their release in the brain. Vitamin C is a key cofactor in the conversion of dopamine to noradrenaline, which I already wrote about that its deficiency is associated with depression, and it is also involved in the regulation of catecholamine and acetylcholine release from synaptic vesicles (both are important neurotransmitters). Another important feature of vitamin C is its antioxidant capacity, and therefore, as already mentioned, its ability to protect the brain. There are studies that clearly indicate that probably every person struggling with depression should consider vitamin C supplementation.

Gariballa S. **Poor vitamin C status is associated with increased depression symptoms following acute illness in older people.** Int J Vitam Nutr Res. 2014;84(1-2):12-7. doi: 10.1024/0300-9831/a000188. PMID: 25835231.

In this randomized, double blind, placebo-controlled trial, scientists investigated the frequency of occurrence of depression symptoms in patients with vitamin C deficiency and normal levels. 322 previously hospitalized acutely-ill older patients were included in the study. Parameters were measured at baseline as well as after 6 weeks and 6 months. At the beginning of the study, vitamin C levels below 11 μmol/L were present in 36% of patients. After six weeks, this level was found in 22% of patients, and after 6 months, 28%. As it turned out, people with low vitamin C levels had a significantly increased risk of symptoms of depression compared with those with higher levels at baseline and at 6 weeks. The authors concluded: "A high proportion of older patients had suboptimal vitamin C status and this was associated with increased symptoms of depression."

Amr, Mostafa et al. **"Efficacy of vitamin C as an adjunct to fluoxetine therapy in pediatric major depressive disorder: a randomized, double-blind, placebo-controlled pilot study."** Nutrition Journal 12 (2013): 31 - 31.

The purpose of this randomized, double-blind, placebo-controlled pilot study was to examine the effect of vitamin C as an adjuvant agent in the treatment of pediatric major depressive disorder. The first group of 12 study participants received fluoxetine (10-20 mg/day) and vitamin C (1 gram/day). The second group of 12 participants also received fluoxetine (10-20 mg/day) but plus placebo. The treatment lasted 6 months. After this time, researchers found that fluoxetine and vitamin C supplementation caused a significant decrease in depressive symptoms compared to fluoxetine plus placebo group as measured by the Children's Depression Rating Scale (CDRS) and Children's Depression Inventory (CDI).

Wang, Yifan et al. **"Effects of vitamin C and vitamin D administration on mood and distress in acutely hospitalized patients 1 – 4."** (2013).

In another randomized, double-blind, active-control clinical trial, the authors investigated the effect of vitamin C supplementation on mood and psychological distress. 75% of acutely hospitalized patients had subnormal plasma total vitamin C concentrations, and 30% had concentrations below 11.4 μmol/L. These patients were given 500 mg of vitamin C twice daily. Scientists found that treatment with vitamin C was associated with a 71% reduction in mood disturbance (assessed with Profile of Mood States) and a 51% reduction in psychological distress (assessed with Distress Thermometer).

Gautam, Medhavi et al. **"Role of antioxidants in generalised anxiety disorder and depression."** Indian Journal of Psychiatry 54 (2012): 244 - 247.

The authors of this study wanted to find out whether vitamin C, E, and β-carotene levels differ between healthy subjects and patients with generalized anxiety disorder (GAD), and whether supplementation with these vitamins leads to improvement. The levels were compared between 80 subjects (40 patients of GAD, 40 patients suffering from depression) in the age group of 20-60 years with a group of 20 healthy controls. The scientists found that the levels of vitamin C, E, and β-carotene were significantly lower compared to healthy controls. Then the patients were divided into two groups. One group received standard treatment, while the other group received standard treatment and vitamin C (1 gram), vitamin E (800 mg) and β-carotene (600 mg) daily for 6 weeks. A significant reduction in anxiety and depression scores was observed in people who supplemented with these vitamins.

de Oliveira, Ivaldo Jesus Lima et al. **"Effects of Oral Vitamin C Supplementation on Anxiety in Students: A Double-Blind, Randomized, Placebo-Controlled Trial."** Pakistan journal of biological sciences : PJBS 18 1 (2015): 11-8 .

de Olveira, et al, in this randomized, double-blind, placebo-controlled trial investigated the effects of vitamin C on anxiety in high school students. 42 students were given vitamin C in an amount of 500 mg a day or a placebo. The anxiety levels were measured both at the start of the study and after 14 days of intervention (with the Beck Anxiety Inventory). The treatment led to higher plasma vitamin C concentrations that were associated with reduced anxiety levels. Moreover, supplementation of this vitamin had a beneficial effect on the heart rate.

CHAPTER 55:
INFERTILITY

Vitamin C can help with infertility for both women and men. Vitamin C can raise progesterone levels in women, which is very important for maintaining early pregnancy. It can help regulate menstrual cycles as well as ovulation. In addition, this vitamin protects against free radicals that may be the cause of luteal phase defects. Interestingly, when a pregnant woman is deficient in vitamin C, her daughter, already an adult, may also have fertility problems. In the case of a man, in turn, vitamin C may affect the quantity and quality of sperm, and consequently his fertility. Let's look at some studies that prove the above claims.

Akmal, Mohammed et al. **"Improvement in human semen quality after oral supplementation of vitamin C**." Journal of medicinal food 9 3 (2006): 440-2 .

In this study, scientists investigated the effect of vitamin C supplementation on various semen parameters in oligospermic, infertile, otherwise healthy subjects. Thirteen men aged 25-35 years old without genital infection or varicocele participated in the study. These men took 1 gram of vitamin C twice a day for a maximum of two months. The study showed that the men's sperm count increased 58% and sperm motility increased 48% compared to the measurements at the start of the study. In the words of the authors themselves: "This study showed that vitamin C supplementation in infertile men might improve sperm count, sperm motility, and sperm morphology and might have a place as an additional supplement to improve the semen quality towards conception."

Dawson, Earl B. et al. **"Effect of ascorbic acid supplementation on the sperm quality of smokers."** Fertility and sterility 58 5

(1992): 1034-9 .

In this study, in turn, the scientists wanted to examine the effect of vitamin C on sperm quality of heavy smokers. Seventy-five men aged 20 to 35 years were divided into three groups. One group received a placebo, the second group received 200 mg of vitamin C daily, and the third group received 1000 mg of vitamin C daily for a month. There was no improvement in sperm quality in the placebo group. In the case of vitamin C groups, supplementation resulted in an improvement, with the greatest improvement in people receiving 1000 mg of vitamin C daily.

Henmi, Hirofumi et al. "**Effects of ascorbic acid supplementation on serum progesterone levels in patients with a luteal phase defect.**" Fertility and sterility 80 2 (2003): 459-61 .

In this study, scientists aimed to evaluate the effectiveness of vitamin C supplementation in patients with luteal phase defects. 76 patients in the treatment group received 750 mg of vitamin C daily, while the second group of 46 (out of 74, 28 patients were withdrawn) did not receive treatment. In the control group, 22% of patients had improvement in progesterone levels, whereas in the group supplementing vitamin C it was 53%. Additionally, 25% of patients in the vitamin C supplementation group and 11% of patients in the untreated group became clinically pregnant. Thus, in conclusion, vitamin C led to a significant increase in the serum progesterone levels in patients with luteal phase defect and in connection helped in getting pregnant.

CHAPTER 56:
BONE HEALTH

Vitamin C, like the already mentioned vitamin D, is essential for bone health. Vitamin C is necessary for collagen synthesis and osteoblastogenesis (production of osteoblasts which are responsible for new bone formation). Vitamin C can prevent the loss of osteoblast differentiation markers, as well as reduce bone loss and stimulate bone formation. On the other hand, a deficiency of this vitamin may stimulate osteoclastogenesis (the production of osteoclasts that degrade bones for resorptive purposes). The benefits of vitamin C supplementation relate to, among others, bone mineral density, risk of fractures and osteoporosis.

Bates CJ. **Vitamin C deficiency in guinea pigs: variable sensitivity of collagen at different sites.** Int J Vitam Nutr Res. 1979;49(1):77-86. PMID: 447454.

In this study, scientists measured collagen synthesis in several tissues in vitamin C-deficient guinea pigs. Of all the tissues examined, vitamin C deficiency had the greatest impact on skin collagen. However, bones were in second place as the tissue most affected by deficiency of this vitamin.

Morton, Deborah J. et al. **"Vitamin C Supplement Use and Bone Mineral Density in Postmenopausal Women."** Journal of Bone and Mineral Research 16 (2001): n. pag.

The purpose of this study was to evaluate the effect of daily vitamin C supplementation on bone mineral density (BMD) in a population-based sample of postmenopausal women. In a study of nearly 1,000 women from a community-based cohort, 277 regularly supplemented with vitamin C. Vitamin C doses varied from 100 mg to 5000 mg per day, although the mean dose was 745 mg. 85% of these participants had been taking vitamin C supplements for more than 3 years. Then, analysis of the measurement results showed that those who supplemented with vitamin C had BMD levels approximately 3% higher at the midshaft radius, femoral neck, and total hip.

Malmir, Hanieh et al. **"Vitamin C intake in relation to bone mineral density and risk of hip fracture and osteoporosis: a systematic review and meta-analysis of observational studies."** British Journal of Nutrition 119 (2018): 847 - 858.

The authors of this publication investigated the association between vitamin C intake and bone mineral density (BMD), risk of fractures and osteoporosis. They analyzed thirty-eight studies involving 106 741 individuals aged 20-103 years in this meta-analysis. As it turned out, higher dietary intakes of vitamin C were significantly associated with BMD. For both men and women, higher vitamin C intakes were associated with a 29% decrease in incidence of hip fracture. In the case of people over the age of 70, this relationship was also significant and the risk was reduced by 28%. Moreover, also in the case of osteoporosis, there was a significant inverse association between vitamin C intake and the incidence of this disease. People who consumed the highest amounts of vitamin C had a 33% reduced risk of osteoporosis.

Sun, Y. et al. **"Dietary vitamin C intake and the risk of hip fracture: a dose-response meta-analysis."** Osteoporosis International 29 (2017): 79-87.

The aim of this meta-analysis was to evaluate the association between the dietary vitamin C intake and the risk of hip fracture. The scientists analyzed six studies involving 7908 controls with 2899 cases of hip fracture. They found a statistically significant correlation between vitamin C intake and the risk of hip fracture. For those with the highest vitamin C intake, the risk was reduced by 27%. Furthermore, the authors of this publication also found a linear dose-response association. Each 50 mg/day increase in vitamin C intake was associated with a 5% reduction in the risk of hip fracture.

CHAPTER 57:
CATARACTS

A high intake of vitamin C may be associated with a lower risk of developing cataracts in the future. This is probably related, again, to the antioxidant properties of vitamin C. Several studies have found a relationship between lens cataract and oxidative damage, i.e. an excessive amount of free radicals that our vitamin is able to neutralize.

Wei, L., Liang, G., Cai, C., & Lv, J. (2016). **Association of vitamin C with the risk of age-related cataract: a meta-analysis**. Acta Ophthalmologica, 94.

Wei, Liang, et al, this meta-analysis investigated the association between vitamin C and the risk of age-related cataract. They analyzed 15 articles with 20 studies for vitamin C intake and eight articles with 10 studies for serum ascorbate. Participants who consumed the highest amounts of vitamin C had a 19% lower risk of age-related cataract than those who consumed the lowest amounts of the vitamin. In addition, the inverse association also applied to nuclear cataract and posterior subcapsular cataract.

CHAPTER 58: SPORT

Studies have also shown that vitamin C supplementation may be beneficial for various parameters related to sport, especially in people with a deficiency of this vitamin.

Bryer, Scott C. and Allan H. Goldfarb. **"Effect of high dose vitamin C supplementation on muscle soreness, damage, function, and oxidative stress to eccentric exercise."** International journal of sport nutrition and exercise metabolism 16 3 (2006): 270-80 .

The authors of this publication examined whether vitamin C before and after eccentric exercise could reduce muscle soreness (MS), oxidative stress, and muscle function. Eighteen healthy men were divided into the vitamin C group and the placebo group. These subjects were either given 3 grams of vitamin C per day or placebo for 2 weeks prior and 4 days after performing 70 eccentric elbow extensions with their non-dominant arm. Muscle soreness increased in both groups, but decreased significantly over the 24 hours in the vitamin C supplementation group. Vitamin C attenuated also the creatine kinase (high levels may indicate muscle injury). Moreover, in contrast to the placebo group, there was no significant increase in the glutathione ratio (oxidized glutathione/total glutathione) in the vitamin C group.

Paschalis, Vassilis et al. **"Low vitamin C values are linked with decreased physical performance and increased oxidative stress: reversal by vitamin C supplementation."** European Journal of Nutrition 55 (2014): 45-53.

Paschalis, Vassilis, et al, investigated the relationship between vitamin C and physical performance and increased oxidative stress. They measured vitamin C levels in 100 men. From this group of men, they then included 10 men with the lowest levels of vitamin C and 10 men with the highest levels of vitamin C. Participants performed aerobic exercise before and after vitamin C supplementation for 30 days. The scientists found that participants with low vitamin C levels had lower VO2 max (body's maximal ability to absorb oxygen during maximum physical exertion) levels compared to the high vitamin C group. They concluded the study: "We show for the first time that low vitamin C concentration is linked with decreased physical performance and increased oxidative stress and that vitamin C supplementation decreases oxidative stress and might increase exercise performance only in those with low initial concentration of vitamin C."

Young, J F et al. **"Green tea extract only affects markers of oxidative status postprandially: lasting antioxidant effect of flavonoid-free diet**[*]**."** British Journal of Nutrition 87 (2002): 343 - 355.

Someone may ask why vitamin C supplementation in a previous study reduced oxidative stress only in those with initial low levels of this vitamin. I'll try to explain it briefly. As with anything, excess can be unfavorable, and this applies to antioxidants (scavenging ROS) as well. As it turns out, low levels of reactive oxygen species (ROS) have been proposed as triggers of an adaptive response that strengthens cellular defensive mechanisms also leading to mitochondrial homeostasis and metabolic balance. This phenomenon is called mitohormesis. An excellent example comes from an extremely well-designed study in which participants were cut off from fruits and vegetables (sources of antioxidants). Such results were not expected by anyone at the time: "The overall effect of the 10-week period without dietary fruits and vegetables was a decrease in oxidative damage to DNA, blood proteins, and plasma lipids, concomitantly with marked changes in antioxidative defence." This is why we have so many reports of serious remissions of many diseases after limiting the consumption of various plants as well as why our vitamin C in large, gram quantities will work best in cases of illness, especially acute ones (e.g. infections).

CHAPTER 59: GOUT

Gout is a common form of inflammatory arthritis. Many studies have shown that vitamin C is able to significantly reduce the risk of this ailment. This is due to the fact that vitamin C has the ability to reduce serum uric acid, which at a high level contributes to the formation of gout.

Choi, Hyon K. et al. **"Vitamin C intake and the risk of gout in men: a prospective study."** Archives of internal medicine 169 5 (2009): 502-7 .

The authors of this publication assessed the relationship between vitamin C intake and the occurrence of gout. They followed nearly 47000 male participants with no history of gout at baseline for 20 years. The participants' daily intake of vitamin C was determined every 4 years. During the observation period, 1317 incident cases of gout were reported. The scientists found that people who consumed 500 to 999 mg of vitamin C per day had a 17% lower risk of gout than those who consumed less than 250 mg of this vitamin per day. Additionally, for those who consumed 1,000 to 1,499 mg and over 1,500 mg of vitamin C per day, the risk was reduced by 34% and 45%, respectively. The same results were found when comparing people who supplemented vitamin C with those who did not. The authors summarized: "Higher vitamin C intake is independently associated with a lower risk of gout. Supplemental vitamin C intake may be beneficial in the prevention of gout."

Juraschek. (2011). **Effect of oral vitamin C supplementation on serum uric acid: A meta-analysis of randomized controlled trials**. Arthritis Care, 63(9), 1295–1306. https://doi.org/info:doi/

This meta-analysis was designed to evaluate the effect of vitamin C on serum uric acid. Thirteen randomized controlled trials with a total of 556 participants were analyzed. The median dose of vitamin C was 500 mg per day and the median duration of the study was 30 days. Finally, the meta-analysis showed that vitamin C significantly reduces serum uric acid. Mean serum uric acid reduction was -0.35 mg/dl. Additionally, the subgroup analysis showed even greater reduction effects of vitamin C.

CHAPTER 60:
ALLERGIES, BITES

Vitamin C can be extremely effective in reducing symptoms of various types of allergies. It is mainly related to the histamine-reducing effect of vitamin C and the antioxidant properties of this vitamin, preventing oxidative stress. Below, I will briefly present two important publications on this subject, as well as the medical experience of the two doctors already mentioned.

Podoshin, L. et al. **"Treatment of perennial allergic rhinitis with ascorbic acid solution."** Ear, nose, & throat journal 70 1 (1991): 54-5 .

The authors of this publication wanted to investigate the impact of ascorbic acid solution (nasal spray) in patients suffering from perennial allergic rhinitis. 60 patients with allergy symptoms, including sneezing and runny nose, were included in this randomized two-week study. As it turned out, ascorbic acid led to a decrease in symptoms in 74% of treated patients.

Vollbracht, Claudia et al. **"Intravenous vitamin C in the treatment of allergies: an interim subgroup analysis of a long-term observational study."** The Journal of International Medical Research 46 (2018): 3640 - 3655.

This study looked at the effects of intravenous vitamin C on various allergy symptoms. The study included 71 patients with disease-specific (pruritus, rhinitis, restlessness) and nonspecific (fatigue, sleep disorders, depression, and lack of concentration) symptoms. These people received intravenous vitamin C in the amount of 7.5 grams for 2-3 weeks in acute and 11-12 weeks in chronic disease. The mean number of vitamin C infusions was 7 in the acute and 26 in the chronic disease group. During treatment. for disease-specific symptoms the mean sum score (0–9 points) decreased by 4.71 points, and for nonspecific symptoms by 4.84 points. Overall, symptoms improved in 97.1% of the patients.

The aforementioned Dr. Robert Cathcart noticed much earlier that ascorbic acid, taken in an amount of a few grams every two hours, for example, is able to block many allergic reactions. He often mentioned himself as an example with his own seasonal hay fever symptoms. To get rid of these symptoms, he took 16 grams of oral ascorbic acid in several doses over 24 hours under conditions of moderate exposure to pollen.

Clinical Guide to the Use of Vitamin C, Lendon H. Smith. M.D, AscorbateWeb, 1988.

Dr. Klenner, in turn, had many patients with all sorts of bites; of snakes, spiders or insects. He often treated them with vitamin C. As a treatment, Dr. Klenner recommended 350 mg/kg of intravenous vitamin C along with calcium gluconate. Here are two cases from his medical practice:

Case 1. An eighteen-year-old woman came to the doctor twenty minutes after the hornet bite. The patient had shortness of breath, difficulty swallowing and hives on her body. She was given 12 grams of vitamin C intravenously. Within minutes after treatment, her allergic symptoms subsided.

Case 2. A four-year-old girl was bitten by a Highland Moccasin. The girl had severe pain in her leg and soon began vomiting. Dr. Klenner gave her 4 grams of vitamin C intravenously. Within 30 minutes, the girl stopped crying, started laughing and drinking normally. The girl slept well, although she still had a slight fever. Consequently, the doctor gave another 4 grams of vitamin C intravenously and then one more time in the late afternoon. Treatment was successful without any anti-serums.

CHAPTER 61: SKIN

Vitamin C deficiency can manifest itself in slow-healing wounds. This is due to the fact that this vitamin is involved in the formation of collagen. Vitamin C deficiency can be associated with peeling of the skin. Moreover, vitamin C shows some effectiveness against acne. This effectiveness is related to the reduction of inflammation by this vitamin and the aforementioned participation in the formation of collagen.

Ruamrak, C et al. "**Comparison of clinical efficacies of sodium ascorbyl phosphate, retinol and their combination in acne treatment.**" International Journal of Cosmetic Science 31 (2009): n. pag.

Scientists conducted a randomized double-blind study comparing the effectiveness of topical formulations containing 5% sodium ascorbyl phosphate and 0.2% retinol, separately as well as in combination. They found that sodium ascorbyl phosphate reduced the inflammatory lesion by 20.14% and 48.82% within 4 and 8 weeks, respectively. In the case of retinol alone, there was also an improvement in the form of reduction of lesions. However, the combined treatment resulted in the reduction of the inflammatory lesion by 29.28% within 4 weeks and 63.10% within 8 weeks. The combined treatment therefore turned out to be the most effective.

Clinical Guide to the Use of Vitamin C, Lendon H. Smith. M.D, AscorbateWeb, 1988.

Vitamin C can also prevent sunburn. While this has been demonstrated by numerous present studies, Dr Klenner already noticed this effect of vitamin C decades ago. He recommended taking one gram of vitamin C every hour or two during sun exposure to prevent sunburn.

CHAPTER 62:
HEAVY METALS

Vitamin C may increase the excretion of heavy metals, mainly lead. As early as over eighty years ago, it was suggested that vitamin C might be beneficial in treating occupational lead exposure. More recent studies have found that higher vitamin C levels are associated with a decreased prevalence of elevated blood lead levels. The following study in mice also proved the heavy metal detoxifying properties of vitamin C.

Lihm, Hoseob et al. **"Vitamin C modulates lead excretion in rats."** Anatomy & Cell Biology 46 (2013): 239 - 245.

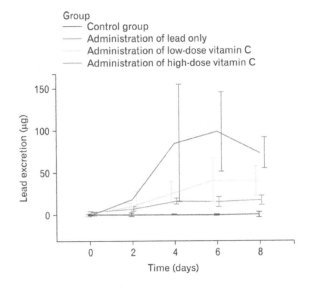

Scientists administered lead orally to 33 mice. Some of the mice also received a lower or higher dose of vitamin C before the intervention. Of the mice that got only lead, 76.9% survived. In the case of mice that received the lower dose of vitamin C, it was 90.9%, whereas in the group with the highest dose of vitamin C, it was 100%. For the group with a low dose of vitamin C (82.43 μg), lead excretion was higher compared to the control group (60.87 μg). However, statistically insignificant. On the other hand, in the group with a high dose of vitamin C, lead excretion (276.13 μg) was significantly higher than in the control group. The body, therefore, thanks to vitamin C was able to excrete much larger amounts of this toxic heavy metal.

CHAPTER 63: OVERALL MORTALITY

Now that we know that vitamin C works on a number of different diseases and conditions, it is worth looking at this vitamin more broadly. Once this is done, it turns out that people who consume more of this vitamin simply live healthier and have a significantly lower risk of all-cause mortality. Unfortunately, we have only observational studies at our disposal, not experimental ones as was often the case in earlier chapters, and thus much less reliable because of the large possible number of other factors.

Loria, Catherine M et al. "**Vitamin C status and mortality in US adults.**" The American journal of clinical nutrition 72 1 (2000): 139-45 .

In this study, scientists investigated the association between serum ascorbate concentrations and mortality. Vitamin C levels were measured as part of the second National Health and Nutrition Examination Survey. The health status was established after 12-16 years. Scientists found that men who had the lowest vitamin C levels (below 28.4 µmol/L) had a 57% higher risk of dying from any cause than those with the highest levels (equal to or greater than 73.8 µmol/L). Additionally, those with the lowest levels compared to those with the highest levels had a 62% greater risk of dying from cancer.

Khaw, Kay-Tee et al. "**Relation between plasma ascorbic acid and mortality in men and women in EPIC-Norfolk prospective study: a prospective population study**." The Lancet 357 (2001): 657-663.

The authors of another study also aimed to investigate the relationship between plasma ascorbic acid and all-cause mortality. 19 496 men and women aged 45-79 years were included in the study. Participants were followed-up for causes of death for about 4 years. People who had the highest plasma ascorbic acid levels had an approximately half lower risk of death than those with the lowest levels of this vitamin. In addition, researchers found that 20 μmol/L rise in plasma ascorbic acid concentration was associated with a 20% reduction in risk of all-cause mortality. This result was independent of age, systolic blood pressure, blood cholesterol, cigarette smoking habit, diabetes, and supplement use.

CHAPTER 64:
SAFETY OF
VITAMIN C

Vitamin C appears to be remarkably safe in both oral and intravenous form. Serious adverse effects occur very rarely, usually in patients with other pre-existing health problems. LD50 (median lethal dose) for humans is unknown. However, for mice, the LD50 is known from experiments and amounts to 11,900 mg/kg of bodyweight. This means that a person weighing, for example, 85 kg would have to get more than 1 kg (1011.5 grams) of vitamin C (at once). When vitamin C is taken orally (in the form of ascorbic acid rather than sodium ascorbate, since the latter is gentler on the stomach), belching, increased bowel movement or loose stools may appear (we know from Dr. Cathcart's publication that the dose should be reduced in case of diarrhea). The most common concerns about vitamin C use include kidney stones, G6PD deficiency, and hemochromatosis. Let's see if these are well-founded concerns.

Matheson, Eric et al. **"Ascorbic Acid Supplements and Kidney Stone Incidence Among Men: A Prospective Study."** (2013).

To investigate the relationship between vitamin C intake and the risk of kidney stones, researchers recruited 48,850 men, aged 45 to 79 years at baseline. People who used supplements other than ascorbic acid were additionally excluded. The observation lasted ten years. During this time, 405 cases of kidney stones were detected in a group of 22,448 people not using vitamin C. In the group of 907 people using vitamin C, there were 31 cases. The study showed that supplementation with ascorbic acid increased the risk of kidney stones by almost 2 times. However, the actual incidence rate was extremely low. The risk of developing kidney stones was 0.16% per year among men who did not supplement with vitamin C and 0.31% per year among those who did. To put it differently, people who did not take vitamin C could get kidney stones every 613.5 years and those who took vitamin C every 322.5 years.

Prier, Melissa et al. "**No Reported Renal Stones with Intravenous Vitamin C Administration: A Prospective Case Series Study.**" Antioxidants 7 (2018): n. pag.

These scientists, in turn, wanted to measure the frequency of reported renal stones in patients receiving intravenous vitamin C therapy. They investigated the cases of 157 adult patients who had this kind of therapy. They found that "No renal stones were reported by any patients in the study, despite 8% of the patients having a history of renal stones. In addition, the majority of patients investigated had stable renal function during the study period as evidenced by little change in serum creatinine levels and estimated glomerular filtration rate (eGFR) following IVC. In conclusion, IVC therapy was not associated with patient-reported renal stones."

In conclusion, there is ample scientific evidence that multigram oral vitamin C supplementation or administration of vitamin C via intravenous infusions is very unlikely to cause renal stone. However, care should be taken in case of renal insufficiency.

People with a deficiency in the enzyme glucose-6-phosphate dehydrogenase are at risk of hemolysis when given high doses of vitamin C. However, such effects have been observed with doses above 40 grams of intravenous vitamin C. Dr Ron Hunninghake of the Riordan Clinic Research Institute, in turn, suggested moderate doses of intravenous vitamin C (25 grams) appear to be safe for people with G6PD deficiency. Nevertheless, red blood cell G6PD levels should be checked before starting intravenous vitamin C therapy.

There is a theory that vitamin C in high doses is not recommended in people with hemochromatosis. This is due to the fact that vitamin C increases the bioavailability of iron. In that case, there could be an "iron overload". However, such cases are rare. There is a lack of good-quality evidence to support this. Even so, caution should be exercised and iron levels monitored during intravenous vitamin C therapy. In the case of high doses of oral vitamin C, it should be taken between meals.

CHAPTER 65:
DETERMINING THE
OPTIMAL DOSE
Who needs more

In order to determine what an adequate intake of vitamin C should be for a person, there are a few things to consider first. Does the person have any disease and is it a serious disease? Does the person use a variety of medical procedures? Does this person drink alcohol or smoke cigarettes? Is it a pregnant woman? These are probably the most important questions. Hope everything will be clear in a moment.

Gan, R., Eintracht, S., & Hoffer, L.J. (2008). **Vitamin C deficiency in a university teaching hospital.** The FASEB Journal, 21.

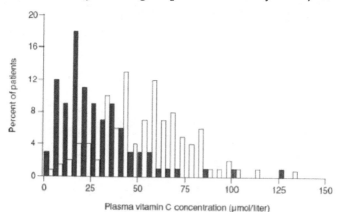

In this publication, the researchers compared the concentrations of vitamin C in hospitalized patients with those of healthy people. In the case of healthy people, subnormal vitamin C concentrations (below 28.4 µmol/L) were present in 13% and deficiency (below 11.4 µmol/L) in 3%. On the other hand, in the group of hospitalized patients, 60% of them had subnormal vitamin C concentrations and 19% were deficient. This significant difference can be clearly seen in the diagram (black bars reflect hospitalized patients).

Adapted from: McGregor & Biesalki, Curr Opin Clin Nutr Metab Care, 2006.

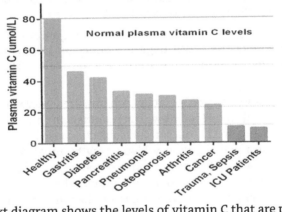

The next diagram shows the levels of vitamin C that are present in people in the cases of particular diseases. As we can see, these are levels well below normal levels in healthy people. Vitamin C levels in people with sepsis or in the intensive care unit are even close to scurvy. These data indicate that people with all these diseases probably need much higher amounts of vitamin C than healthy people, because their bodies use much more of this vitamin and that they should consider supplementing with vitamin C.

The situation similar to the above, obviously also applies to many other diseases (if not all). In addition, it is worth noting that not only they (diseases) affect vitamin C levels, but also the procedures associated with them. An example is dialysis in patients with chronic renal failure. Also, various surgeries significantly reduce the amount of vitamin C in the body. Some doctors recommend giving this vitamin prior to such a procedure.

Many studies have also shown that smokers have lower levels of vitamin C. Naturally, the more cigarettes a day, the lower the concentration will be. This concentration may be up to 30-40% lower compared to non-smokers. One cigarette has been estimated to destroy approximately 25 mg of vitamin C. Therefore, it makes sense that smokers often need much more vitamin C than non-smokers, especially when they smoke a dozen or so cigarettes a day. What's also interesting, vitamin C can prevent angina chest pain when given at a higher dose. This has been proven by scientists in the study below.

Zhang J , Ying X , Lu Q , et al : **A single high dose of vitamin C counteracts the acute negative effect on microcirculation induced by smoking a cigarette**. Microvasc Res 58:305-311, 1999.

Cigarette smoking is associated with impaired microcirculation, including reduced blood flow. The scientists in this study found that smoking in 23 out of 24 subjects caused a significant decrease in microcirculatory blood flow by up to 40-50% (1-5 min after smoking). They also proved that vitamin C can prevent this. Vitamin C in the amount of 2 grams administered 2 hours before smoking reduced this negative phenomenon induced by cigarettes by over 50%. It is also worth adding that only 1 gram of vitamin C did not have such a significant preventive effect.

Faizallah, R M et al. "**Alcohol enhances vitamin C excretion in the urine.**" Alcohol and alcoholism 21 1 (1986): 81-4 .

A higher intake of vitamin C also seems to be adequate for people who drink alcohol regularly. This is because alcohol increases urinary vitamin C losses. In the above study, ascorbic acid excretion was measured in 9 male volunteers four hours before and after administration of, among others, whiskey and lager. Alcohol in either form increased urinary ascorbic acid excretion by 47% in these people.

People who are on high-carbohydrate diets will also require higher amounts of vitamin C. This is related to what I said in the diabetes chapter. Dehydroascorbate (oxidized ascorbate), enters cells via glucose transporter. Therefore, dehydroascorbate and glucose compete with each other. High glucose levels will not just allow vitamin C to enter the cell. This also seems to be the main reason why people who consume almost no carbohydrates but also very small amounts of vitamin C, such as those on the carnivore diet, do not get scurvy.

When pregnant, the body also needs more vitamin C. This is essential for the proper development of the baby. As it turns out, the baby, placenta, and cord contain twice as much vitamin C as is present in maternal blood. Moreover, there is three times more vitamin C in the amniotic fluid than in the mother's blood. Of course, this vitamin C is necessary for the formation of skin, bones, cartilage, etc., but there is another interesting aspect that I will just mention. About 60% of babies develop jaundice. This is due to an excess of bilirubin. About 5% of babies have bilirubin levels so high that it requires treatment. Many doctors claim from their own medical practice that this can be prevented to some extent with vitamin C.

Abdul-Razzak, Khalid K et al. "**Antioxidant vitamins and hyperbilirubinemia in neonates**." GMS German Medical Science 5 (2007): n. pag.

Parameters	Neonates without hyperbilirubinemia (n=119)		Neonates with hyperbilirubinemia (n=11)		P value (95% CI)
	Mean (SD)	Median (Range)	Mean (SD)	Median (Range)	
Vitamin C (µmol/l)	132 (36)	127.7 (56-250)	87 (22)	89.4 (62-124)	0.0001 (0.4500,1.0501)
Vitamin E (µmol/l)	10.4 (5)	9.1 (4-40)	7.5 (2)	6.3 (5-14.8)	0.001 (0.500,1.700)
Bilirubin (µmol/l)	65 (24)	58.1 (15-100)	238 (56)	246.2 (143-306)	0.0001 (-12.400,-8.370)

The authors of this publication investigated the relationship between plasma vitamin C and E levels and the severity of hyperbilirubinemia in full-term neonates. They found that both vitamin C and vitamin E levels were significantly lower in children with hyperbilirubinemia. As you can see in the table, in babies with hyperbilirubinemia the average vitamin C level is

87 μmol/L, while in babies without hyperbilirubinemia it is over 130 μmol/L. This suggests a possible link between this condition and vitamin C.

How is it in animals and what doses were recommended by respected doctors

A large proportion of animals produce their own vitamin C. Guinea pigs, fruit bats, primates, and obviously humans are exceptions. It is caused by the enzyme L-Gulonolactone oxidase, which is not active in them (and us). This enzyme allows the conversion of glucose to ascorbic acid. The exact reason for this malfunction is not fully known. However, as a consequence, we have to take care of vitamin C intake ourselves to be able to function at all.

Producing vitamin C	Not producing vitamin C
Cow: 18 mg/kg/day + food	Guinea pig: 20-33 mg/kg/day (from food)
Cat: 20-40 mg/kg/day	Gorilla: 30 mg/kg/day (from food)
Goat: 185 mg/kg/day (and 1400 mg/kg/day in case of illness)	Human: 1.2 mg/kg/day (RDA)

The table above shows the amount of vitamin C produced by each individual animal (first column) as well as the amount of vitamin C consumed in nature (second column). Humans are also added to the table along with their recommended daily intake of vitamin C. The first important thing is that, as we can see, all the animals mentioned above produce/consume significantly more vitamin C per kg of body weight than is recommended for humans. For example, if we calculate this, our cat can produce twice as much vitamin C than is recommended for humans. Goats even much more. Interestingly, in the case of disease, the production of vitamin C in goats increases several times. And unsurprisingly, goats are known to be animals that rarely get sick. Gorillas, on the other hand, do not produce vitamin C and must consume it from food. They eat approximately 30 mg/kg/

day of vitamin C, which is 4,000-6700 mg of this vitamin per day depending on the weight of the animal. If the gorilla's weight was the same as that of a human (e.g. 80 kg), the vitamin C intake would be probably 2400 mg. The same could be the case with guinea pigs. Meanwhile, the recommended amount for an adult male is about only 90 mg of vitamin C per day. While animals are not perfect evidence of how much vitamin C is required for humans, they can be a good clue. It is worth taking this into account.

NOTE: Natural and synthetic ascorbic acid (vitamin C) are chemically identical. Human studies have shown no difference in biological activity between them. The only difference not related to health is the much higher price of this of natural origin.

At this point, I would also like to present what amounts of vitamin C were recommended by well-known and respected doctors researching the topic of vitamin C, without whose work this book could not have been written:
  - Dr Frederick Klenner: 10 grams
  - Dr Linus Pauling: 2.3 to 9 grams
  - Dr Robert F. Cathcart: 4 to 15 grams (depending on bowel tolerance)
  - Dr Irwin Stone: 70 mg/kg/day
  - Dr Steve Hickey: 500 mg to 20 grams (depending on current health)
  - Dr Matthias Rath: 600 mg to 3 grams
  - Dr Thomas Levy: 3 to 9 grams
  - Dr Suzanne Humphries: 200 mg to 1 gram (from food but in the absence of disease or stress)

Importantly, the above recommendations probably apply mainly to ordinary people who neither limit carbohydrate intake in their diets nor are perfectly healthy.

PART III: IODINE

CHAPTER 66:
CANCER

Zava, T.T., & Zava, D.T. (2011). **Assessment of Japanese iodine intake based on seaweed consumption in Japan: A literature-based analysis.** Thyroid Research, 4, 14 - 14.

It is well known that the Japanese have one of the highest intakes of iodine in the world. This is mainly due to the high consumption of seaweeds, which are rich in this element. However, it is not easy to estimate exactly how much iodine the Japanese actually consume as it differs from generation to generation and region to region. The authors of the above publication have just undertaken this task. After a long analysis, they concluded that the Japanese iodine intake largely from seaweeds averages 1-3 mg/day. For example, the Recommended Dietary Allowance (RDA) for adult men and women is only 150 µg/day. So these are amounts that are at least 6.7 to 20 times less than what the Japanese consume on a daily basis. The authors of this publication also mentioned several possible associations between seaweeds and iodine consumption and the unique health statistics of the Japanese. First, the Japanese have one of the highest life expectancy, almost 6 years longer than that of the US. Infant mortality in 2004 was more than twice as high in the USA as in Japan (6.8 vs 2.8/100,000). In 1999, the death rate associated with breast cancer was more than three times higher in the US than in Japan. However, the breast cancer incidence rate increased in Japanese immigrants who had emigrated to the US. In addition, in 2002, the rate of prostate cancer in Japanese was 12.6 per 100,000 and was almost ten times lower than in the United States. As I hope the next chapter on cancer and iodine will show, this statistic is probably not aleatory.

Kargar, Saeed et al. "**Urinary Iodine Concentrations in Cancer Patients.**" Asian Pacific Journal Cancer Prevention : APJCP 18

(2017): 819 - 821.

To begin with, before we move on to the different types of cancer, there is one thing that they all have in common. Namely, they accompany iodine deficiencies. The authors of this publication have confirmed this. They examined iodine levels in 85 Iranian patients diagnosed with different types of cancer. They found that the median urinary iodine concentration was 17.4 µg/L indicating severe deficiency. Overall, 88.1% had severe iodine deficiency (<20 µg/L), 7.1% moderate iodine deficiency (20-49 µg/L), and 2.4% mild deficiency (50-99 µg/L). Thus, only 2.4% of patients had sufficient levels according to the WHO/UNICEF/ICCIDD classification.

Thyroid cancer

ISLER H. **Effect of iodine on thyroid tumors induced in the rat by a low-iodine diet**. J Natl Cancer Inst. 1959 Oct;23:675-93. PMID: 14405943.

More than 60 years ago, Dr. Isler showed in rats that iodine deficiency can lead to thyroid cancer. Rats were on a low-iodine diet which resulted in neoplastic thyroid nodules. After this time they received an iodine supplement. Iodine supplementation resulted in reappearance of thyroid hormone in the blood and normalization of the level of thyrotropic hormone. Furthermore, iodine caused a regression in the size of the thyroid gland.

Schaller Jr RT, Stevenson JK. **Development of carcinoma of the thyroid in iodine-deficient mice**. Cancer. 1966;19:1063–80.

Other scientists conducted a similar study on rats with similar effects. Within 6 to 12 months of iodine deficiency, 78% (61/78) of mice experienced extreme hypertrophy and hyperplasia of the thyroid. In another eleven of them, the thyroid morphology indicated papillary adenocarcinoma. Additionally, after 18 months, necropsy in 8 of 30 mice revealed malignant neoplasms of the thyroid. Overall, the initial hyperplasia of the thyroid turned into nodular over time. The cysts then emerged and papillary hyperplasia developed. Sometimes it ended with a malignant change. Importantly, these abnormalities proved to be completely reversible up to 9 months when the mice were additionally supplemented with potassium iodide.

Correa P, Welsh RA. **The effect of excessive iodine intake on the thyroid gland of the rat.** Arch Pathol. 1960;70:247–51.

On the other hand, the authors of this publication investigated the effects of excessive iodine doses on the thyroid gland of the rats. Sprague Dawley male rats were given 119 mg of potassium iodide along with the daily diet for 9 months. Iodine caused a significant increase in thyroid weight as well as some histologic changes. However, scientists found no evidence of a reduction in thyroid function. Moreover, thyroid tumors were also not observed.

Liu, Zhiting and Ai-hua Lin. **"Dietary Factors and Thyroid Cancer Risk: A Meta-Analysis of Observational Studies."** Nutrition and Cancer 66 (2014): 1165 - 1178.

In this meta-analysis of 19 observational studies, scientists examined the relationship between dietary factors and thyroid cancer incidence. They analyzed the highest and lowest consumption of fish, vegetables, shellfish, cruciferous vegetables, fruits, meat and grain, and the risk of thyroid cancer in different populations. Overall, the highest fish consumption was associated with a 21% reduction in thyroid cancer risk. Naturally, fish is also one of the main sources of iodine for humans. The results for the other dietary factors were insignificant. In addition, subgroup analysis showed that the highest consumption of fish and shellfish reduced the risk of thyroid cancer by 26 and 54%, respectively. These results were for populations in iodine-poor regions.

Cardis E, Kesminiene A, Ivanov V, Malakhova I, Shibata Y, Khrouch V, et al. **Risk of thyroid cancer after exposure to 131I in childhood.** J Natl Cancer Inst. 2005;97:724–32.

As for radioactivity. The Chernobyl nuclear accident from April 1986 resulted in an increase in incidence of childhood thyroid cancer in radioactively contaminated areas. The iodine 131I isotope was responsible for this. Therefore, a group of scientists decided to specifically evaluate the risk of thyroid cancer after exposure to 131I as well as investigate other promoting factors.

They studied 276 case patients with thyroid cancer and 1300 matched control subjects. All of these people were under 15 at the time of the nuclear power plant accident. Scientists observed a strong link between radiation dose received and thyroid cancer risk. It was even a linear dose-response relationship up to 1.5-2 Gy. As it turned out, in iodine-deficient areas, the risk of radiation-related thyroid cancer was also more than three times greater than elsewhere. Furthermore, scientists calculated that potassium iodide supplementation reduced the risk of radiation-related thyroid cancer by a factor of 3. That is why, in Poland, after the Chernobyl catastrophe, children and adolescents began to be massively given Lugol's solution. This was to prevent the entry of iodine 131I into the thyroid gland and its serious consequences.

Gastric cancer

Gulaboglu, Mine et al. **"Comparison of iodine contents in gastric cancer and surrounding normal tissues."** Clinical Chemistry and Laboratory Medicine (CCLM) 43 (2005): 581 - 584.

Many studies have suggested that iodine is also linked to gastric cancer. One of them is the Turkish one above. Among cancers, stomach cancer ranked first in the north-eastern Anatolia region (Turkey). This region was known for common iodine deficiency. To study this topic, Turkish scientists decided to determine iodine levels in gastric cancer and surrounding normal tissues in 19 patients with gastric cancer. They found that tissue iodine levels were significantly lower in gastric cancer tissue (17.8+/-3.4 ng I/mg protein) than in surrounding normal tissue (41.7+/-8.0 ng I/mg protein). They concluded: "The iodine deficiency in our region may be one of the factors for increased gastric cancer prevalence. Our results support the hypothesis that iodine plays an important role in gastric cancer development."

Behrouzian R, Aghdami N. **Urinary iodine/creatinine ratio in patients with stomach cancer in Urmia, Islamic Republic of Iran.** *East Mediterr Health J.* 2004;10:921-4.

Iranian authors of the above publication also investigated the relationship between iodine deficiency and stomach cancer. They included 100 patients diagnosed with stomach cancer and 84 healthy people (control group) in whom they measured the ratio of urinary iodine to urinary creatinine. Mean urinary iodine levels in gastric cancer patients (61.9 μg/g creatinine) were significantly lower than in the control group (101.7 μg/g creatinine). Moreover, severe iodine deficiency (below 25 μg/g creatinine) affected 49% of people with gastric cancer and 19.1% of people in the control group.

Scientists also observed something else related to stomach cancer and NIS. The sodium/iodide symporter (NIS) is an integral plasma membrane glycoprotein that mediates iodide transport in the thyroid, salivary glands, lactating breasts and stomach. Namely, scientists noted that NIS expression is significantly limited or even absent in gastric cancer. This is not favorable, which I will mention later in the book.

Breast cancer

Aceves, Carmen et al. **"Is Iodine A Gatekeeper of the Integrity of the Mammary Gland?"** Journal of Mammary Gland Biology and Neoplasia 10 (2005): 189-196.

As I just wrote, iodine is taken up by the sodium/iodide symporter (NIS) in the breasts. There iodine plays an important role contributing to the normal growth of breast tissue and to the integrity of the mammary gland. High iodine intake (up to 25 times greater than in Western countries) has been linked to the low incidence of breast cancer in Japanese women. In addition, the authors of this publication mentioned that in animal models, iodine in the form of a supplement or seaweed has been shown to inhibit breast cancer cells and tumor growth. They proposed that iodine should be considered as an adjuvant in breast cancer therapy.

Funahashi, Hiroomi et al. **"Seaweed Prevents Breast Cancer?"** Japanese Journal of Cancer Research : Gann 92 (2001): 483 - 487.

The study I posted above is one that investigated the chemopreventive effects of seaweed on breast cancer. These scientists earlier had found that wakame (a type of seaweed) has a suppressive effect on rat mammary tumors, possibly by inducing apoptosis (programmed death of cancer cells). In the present study, in turn, they used seaweed mekabu, which they administered to rats in daily drinking water. This iodine-rich seaweed "showed an extremely strong suppressive effect on rat mammary carcinogenesis". Additionally, in vitro, mekabu solution strongly induced apoptosis in three kinds of human breast cancer cells. The effect of this seaweed turned out to be even stronger than the chemotherapeutic agent known and commonly used in breast cancer.

As for still animal studies on the effects of iodine on breast cancer. Several others also showed that iodine (this time not from seaweed) in high concentrations reduces the occurrence of mammary cancer induced chemically in rats.

Yang, Yoon Jung et al. "**A case–control study on seaweed consumption and the risk of breast cancer.**" British Journal of Nutrition 103 (2009): 1345 - 1353.

Gim and miyeok are some of the most popular and consumed seaweeds in South Korea. They are also the main source of iodine in Korean people. The authors of this publication from Hanyang University investigated the association between the intake of these seaweeds and the risk of breast cancer. 362 women aged 30-65 years old with histologically confirmed breast cancer were included in the study. The scientists also estimated the food intake of these people. They found that the mean intake of gim in people with breast cancer was lower than in the control group. The daily intake of gim was inversely associated with the risk of breast cancer. People with the highest gim consumption (5th quintile) had a 52% lower risk of breast cancer than those with the lowest gim consumption (1st quintile).

Stoddard FR 2nd, Brooks AD, Eskin BA, Johannes GJ. **Iodine alters gene expression in the MCF7 breast cancer cell line: evidence for an anti-estrogen effect of iodine.** Int J Med Sci. 2008;5(4):189-96.

Due to the laboratory evidence that iodine may inhibit cancer growth through modulation of the estrogen pathway, Stoddard and colleagues decided to investigate this topic in more detail.

They analyzed the effect of Lugol's iodine solution (5% iodine, 10% potassium iodide) on gene expression in the estrogen responsive breast cancer cell line. Analysis showed 29 genes that were up-regulated and 14 genes that were down-regulated in response to Lugol's iodine solution treatment. These changes concerned genes related to hormone metabolism, regulation of cell cycle growth and differentiation. For example, iodine/iodide treatment increased BRCA1 activity. BRCA1 protein is known to regulate estrogen signaling in the breast. Moreover, individuals with mutations in BRCA1 are at an increased risk of breast cancers. Potentially, those effects on genes may be important in the prevention or treatment of breast cancer. The authors summarized this study with these words: "In addition to elucidating our understanding of the effects of iodine/iodide on breast cancer, this work suggests that iodide/iodide may be useful as an adjuvant therapy in the pharmacologic manipulation of the estrogen pathway in women with breast cancer."

Dr. Jonathan Wright also reported that iodine in the form of Lugol's solution can help maintain proper levels between estrogens (estrone, estradiol and estriol), promoting estriol production as well. Higher levels of estradiol and estrone have been linked to a higher risk of developing breast cancer. Moreover, some animal studies have also suggested a preventive effect of estriol in breast cancer.

Nuñez-Anita, Rosa Elvira et al. **"Peroxisome proliferator-activated receptors: role of isoform gamma in the antineoplastic effect of iodine in mammary cancer."** Current cancer drug targets 11 7 (2011): 775-86 .

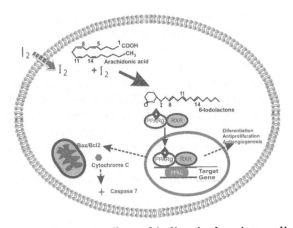

The strong anti-cancer effect of iodine is due, inter alia, to 6-iodolactone. 6-iodolactone is one of the iodinated lipids that is formed from iodine and arachidonic acid with the participation of TPO (as seen above). This lipid has an antiproliferative and apoptotic effect on various types of cancer, including breast, colorectal, prostate and thyroid cancer. Thus, simple iodine supplementation can play an extremely important role in the prevention and treatment of cancer. However, for 6-iodolactone to be formed, iodine concentrations must be higher. Scientists found the presence of 6-iodolactone in people whose daily iodine intake was 15 mg. Therefore, we can assume that doses equal to and greater than 15 mg per day will be appropriate for those who care about the formation of 6-iodolactone. On the other hand, this lipid cannot be detected in the tissues of people who are iodine deficient. The recommended dose of 150 μg does not contribute to this either.

Aceves, Carmen et al. **"The extrathyronine actions of iodine as antioxidant, apoptotic, and differentiation factor in various tissues."** Thyroid : official journal of the American Thyroid Association 23 8 (2013): 938-46 .

The authors of the above scientific study not only pointed to the reports of other researchers that iodine supplements at low (1.5–8 mg/day) and intermediate doses (10–32 mg/day), ingested from a variety of sources, are well-tolerated in euthyroid subjects, maintaining levels of thyroid hormones (T4 and T3) and thyrotropin (TSH) within normal limits but also suggested iodine supplementation recommendations of at least 3 mg/day for pathologies of tissues that take up iodine (primarily thyroid, mammary, and prostate glands and potentially pancreas, gastric, and nervous systems). They justified this with the antioxidant (10- or 50- fold greater than of ascorbic acid and potassium iodide, respectively) and antiproliferative properties of iodine, which exert a suppressive effect on the development and size of both benign and cancerous neoplasias by contributing to apoptosis and the formation of the aforementioned iodolipids.

Prostate cancer

Hoption Cann SA, Qiu Z, van Netten C. **A prospective study of iodine status, thyroid function, and prostate cancer risk: follow-up of the First National Health and Nutrition Examination Survey.** *Nutr Cancer.* 2007;58:28-34.

The authors of this publication wanted to investigate the relationship between iodine status and prostate cancer risk as well as the relationship between thyroid disease and prostate cancer risk. To do this, they analyzed the data from the NHANES I Epidemiologic Follow-up Study. The analysis showed that those with the highest iodine levels had a 29% lower risk of prostate cancer compared with those with the lowest iodine levels. Additionally, people with thyroid disease had more than twice the risk of prostate cancer than people without the disease. And people who were diagnosed with thyroid disease more than 10 years earlier had a risk more than three times higher. Later in the book you will learn that the relationship between iodine and the thyroid gland is also very important.

Aranda N, Sosa S, Delgado G, Aceves C, Anguiano B. **Uptake and antitumoral effects of iodine and 6-iodolactone in differentiated and undifferentiated human prostate cancer cell lines.** *Prostate.* 2013;73:31-41.

There is evidence that iodine treatment is able to inhibit cell proliferation and induce apoptosis in breast cancer and thyroid cancer. In this study, in turn, the scientists wanted to investigate the antiproliferative and apoptotic effects of iodine, iodide and 6-iodolactone in human prostate cell lines. Non-cancerous (RWPE-1), cancerous (LNCaP, DU-145) cells and nude mice xenotransplanted with cancerous DU-145 were used as a cancer model. RWPE-1 cells were most sensitive to iodide and 6-iodolactone, while LNCaP cells to iodine. Both iodine and iodide caused activation of the intrinsic apoptotic pathway in all three cell lines. Moreover, iodine administration impaired growth of the cancerous (DU-145) tumor cells in nude mice. The above results indicated that in order to obtain the best therapeutic effects, it is probably worth using several forms of iodine simultaneously. Even normal Lugol's solution seems to be appropriate. The authors concluded the study: "Normal and cancerous prostate cells can take up iodine, and depending on the chemical form, it exerts antiproliferative and apoptotic effects both in vitro and in vivo."

Anguiano B, et al. **Therapeutic effect of iodine on human benign prostatic hyperplasia.** Paper presented at: 14th International Thyroid Congress. September 11-16, 2010. Paris, France. Abstract ITC2010-2585.

In this study, scientists wanted to evaluate the effects of iodine therapy on prostatic hyperplasia in men. Patients received 5 mg of Lugol's solution per day for 8 months. During this time, scientists observed that the characteristic symptoms of benign prostatic hyperplasia decreased by 30 to 40%. In addition, there were also significant declines in circulating PSA levels. High PSA levels may indicate the presence of prostate cancer. Iodine therapy also improved urinary flow in these patients. Importantly, iodine did not change the levels of T3, T4 and TSH and the patients did not report any general health problems.

Anecdotal evidence
1. The older man struggled with a diseased prostate. He had problems urinating, including pollakiuria. For several months, he increased the daily iodine dose to a final dose of 50 mg per day. Gradually, his prostate-related ailments decreased until after a few months they completely subsided.

CHAPTER 67:
FIBROCYSTIC
BREAST DISEASE

Fibrocystic breast disease is a very common breast condition that affects up to 50% of women between the ages of 20 and 50. It is often associated with symptoms such as breast pain, tenderness and lumpiness that may intensify just before menstruation. Iodine, which some say "loves breasts", is able to get rid of this unpleasant condition. To obtain this effect, as shown by research and medical practice, the dosages used for treatment should be in milligrams. This is mainly due to the fact that iodine plays a significant role in the development and maintenance of healthy breast tissue, and breasts, which require a lot of it.

Ghent, William R Dr et al. **"Iodine replacement in fibrocystic disease of the breast."** *Canadian journal of surgery. Journal canadien de chirurgie* 36 5 (1993): 453-60 .

This study is a review of three clinical studies examining the response of patients with fibrocystic breast disease to iodine replacement therapy. In the first part of the first study, 233 subjects were treated with 5% Lugol's solution for two years. The daily dose of iodine ranged from 31.25 mg to 62.5 mg. 70% of subjects treated had clinical improvement in their fibrocystic breast disease. Changes in thyroid function appeared in 4% of them and symptoms of iodism were present in 3% of them. In the second part of the first study, 588 patients were given 10 mg of caseinate iodine over a 5-year period. In this case, clinical improvements were seen in only 40% of patients. In the first part of the second study 145 patients treated for several months but not yet cured caseinate iodine (still having residual symptoms and signs of fibrocystic breast disease) were switched to aqueous molecular iodine therapy in the amount of 0.08 mg/kg (about 3-6 mg per day). As it turned out, after about 10 months, 74.5% of these patients in the crossover series had clinical improvement, having pain-free breasts. In addition, in a group of 108 patients, iodine therapy resulted in the disappearance of microcysts within 5 months. Objective improvement was experienced by 78.1% of these subjects and 98% were pain-free at evaluation. This study also showed that iodine is more effective than iodide in the case of this ailment. This is due to the fact that the breast tissue concentrates iodine. In turn, for example, the thyroid and salivary glands prefer iodide. I will mention this aspect later. The third prospective double-blind study enrolled 56 patients, of which 23 received between 0.7 and 0.9 mg/kg of iodine (so doses were similar to those in the second study) for six months. In the group treated with iodine, 65% of people had subjective improvement, whereas in the control group it was 33% of people. Moreover, 65% of the subjects had an objective improvement in the iodine group. In contrast, there was a 3% objective deterioration in the control group. The side effects of iodine treatment (from the second study with a total of 1,365 patients treated) were minor. For example: nausea was reported in 0.6% of patients, hyperthyroidism in 0.1%, hypothyroidism in 0.3%, and headache in 0.2%. Increased breast pain was the most commonly reported side effect, affecting 5.7% of patients. However, this pain was short-lived and possibly related to softening of the breast and disappearance of fibrous tissue plaques.

Kessler, J. (2004). **The Effect of Supraphysiologic Levels of Iodine on Patients with Cyclic Mastalgia.** The Breast Journal, 10.

Sometime later, Kessler conducted a randomized, double-blind, placebo-controlled trial involving 111 otherwise healthy euthyroid women with breast pain. Patients enrolled in the study had moderate or severe breast pain and fibrosis involving at least 25% of both breast surfaces. Tenderness, and nodularity each cycle was also assessed in these women. Patients were given placebo, 1.5 mg, 3 mg, or 6 mg of iodine daily for six months. Reductions in all physician assessments were observed in patients in the 3 mg iodine group and 6 mg iodine group. However, such an effect was not observed in the 1.5 mg iodine group or in the placebo group. Statistically significant decreases in pain were reported in the two groups with higher iodine doses as early as 3 months after initiation of therapy. Furthermore, in the 6 mg iodine group, 50% of patients experienced clinically significant reduction in overall pain. Importantly, no adverse event was observed for each iodine dose.

Flechas, J.D., **Orthoiodosupplementation in a primary care practice**. The Original Internist, 12(2):89-96, 2005.

Dr. Jorge D. Flechas treated 200 women with fibrocystic breast disease over the course of four years. Women who came to him had a mean Ghent score of 15.7 (which includes micronodularity, tenderness, fibrous tissue plaques, macrocysts and turgidity) and an average age of 41.4 years. He found that the mean score after six months of treatment drops to 12.8, 10.2, and 8.6 at iodine doses of 12.5 mg, 25 mg, and 37.5 mg per day, respectively. When receiving 50 mg of iodine, the patient's mean score drops to 7.6 within 3 to 6 months and to 3.8 after one year of treatment. There is also sometimes a score of zero and the disappearance of breast pain in 1 to 30 days at a dose of 50 mg. If symptoms resolved completely, he suggested reducing the iodine intake to 12.5 to 25 mg per day. According to him, 50 mg of iodine per day is the optimal dose for this ailment. In his patients undergoing therapy, he did not observe major changes in serum T4, TSH and free T3.

Importantly, the breasts in the case of this condition can also be smeared with iodine (e.g. Lugol's solution). To avoid irritation, iodine can be mixed with some oil beforehand. As always, regular use brings the best results.

Anecdotal evidence
1. The woman started taking iodine more than a year before. She started with a dose of 6.25 mg of iodine slowly up to 50 mg for several months now. After some time, her breasts stopped being tender and, moreover, her periods stopped being very painful

and became mild.

2. The middle-aged woman suffered from breast lumps. For this reason, she started iodine therapy at 50 mg iodine/iodide tablets per day. After about a quarter of the year, the breasts were soft and did not hurt. In the meantime, her well-being also improved, the woman had more energy and thought more clearly.

CHAPTER 68:
THYROID HEALTH

Goiter

Marine, David and O. P. Kimball. "**PREVENTION OF SIMPLE GOITER IN MAN: FOURTH PAPER.**" *JAMA Internal Medicine* 25: 661-672.

Almost a century ago, David Marine and O. P. Kimball conducted a study investigating the effects of iodine on the prevention and treatment of goiter. Teenage girls between the ages of 10 and 18 from the city of Akron, Ohio, in which the goiter incidence was over 50%, were included in the study. 2,305 girls were placed in the control group and were not given iodine. In turn, 2,190 girls received a total of 4 grams of sodium iodine per year. They were given 0.2 grams of sodium iodine for the consecutive 10 days each spring and fall. This dose is equivalent to about 10 mg per day. As it turned out, at the first examination, 65% of girls who took iodine had a decrease in the size of the thyroid gland. In the control group it was only 14%. Overall, after more than two and a half years of follow-up, 21.5% of girls in the control group developed thyroid enlargement, whereas in the iodine group it was only 0.2%. Symptoms of iodism (for example unpleasant brassy taste, coryza, sneezing, and headache, which however may disappear quickly) affected less than 0.5% of girls. They were usually mild so supplementation could continue.

Clements, F. W.. "**Goitre prophylaxis by addition of potassium iodate to bread. Experience in Tasmania.**" *Lancet* 1 7645 (1970): 489-92 .

More than half a century ago, iodine, as a universal prophylactic against endemic goiter, began to be administered to infants, preschool children and schoolchildren from Tasmania. Children were given tablets containing 10 mg of potassium iodide once a week (equivalent to 1.4 mg per day). During the sixteen years of iodine administration, there was a slow steady reduction in the prevalence of goiter. The exceptions were some regions where there was no such significant reduction in the number of thyroid goiters, which was associated with ineffective distribution of the tablets and/or the occurrence of goitrogens.

Hintze, Gerhard et al. **"Treatment of endemic goitre due to iodine deficiency with iodine, levothyroxine or both: results of a multicentre trial."** European Journal of Clinical Investigation 19 (1989): n. pag.

Researchers have also shown that iodine given to people with goiter may be similarly effective or more effective than administration of levothyroxine alone. They randomized 166 patients into three groups; the first received 150 µg levothyroxine/day, the second 400 µg iodine/day and the third a combination of 75 µg levothyroxine and 200 µg iodine/day. The administration period was 8 months followed by a 4-month break. They documented a significant decrease in goiter size in each of the three groups of -32.1% in the first group, -37.3% in the second and -38.7% in the third. However, unlike the second group where the therapeutic effect was sustained after 4 months of discontinuation of iodine administration, the first group experienced a significant increase in thyroid volume again. In the third group, a slight "rebound effect" was observed, but greater than in the group supplementing iodine alone. Thus, these results indicated that iodine produces the best results in reducing goiter.

Dozens of more recent studies have also shown that goiter is closely related to iodine deficiency, and knowledge in this regard is already fairly common. That is why iodized salt was introduced. For people with urinary iodine concentration below 20 µg/L, the goiter incidence is especially higher. The iodine derived from iodized salt is able to prevent this and increase iodine concentration over these 20 µg/L. However, as has already been seen and will continue to be, iodized salt is not able to provide enough iodine for the proper functioning of the whole organism and protection against many diseases.

Although iodine deficiency in goiter plays a key role, scientists also found other factors that may be involved in the goiter formation process. This is, for example, a deficiency of selenium, iron or vitamin A. Goiter formation can also be promoted by food products such as cassava, lima beans, sweet potato, cruciferous vegetables (cabbage, kale, cauliflower, broccoli) by competing metabolites of certain substances contained in these products with iodine for thyroidal uptake. Similarly for soybeans and millet. Nonetheless, the above products should not be a problem if iodine consumption is adequate.

Thyroid disease

As we already know, severe iodine deficiency is significantly associated with the occurrence of thyroid goiter. Such a deficiency is also associated with hypothyroidism (more on that in a moment). When iodine levels are very low, even though there is an increase in thyroid activity to maximize iodine uptake, the thyroid gland is unable to produce sufficient amounts of thyroid hormones. In cases of mild iodine deficiency, in turn, increased thyroid activity can compensate for low iodine concentration and maintain a relatively normally functioning thyroid gland. However, this chronic thyroid stimulation may contribute to an increased incidence of hyperthyroidism as well as the toxic nodular goiter. Hence, also, as long as iodine levels do not increase in the population, the prevalence of thyroid disease will be high. Many scientific studies prove this.

Weng, Wan-wen et al. **"A PRISMA-compliant systematic review and meta-analysis of the relationship between thyroid disease and different levels of iodine intake in mainland China."** Medicine 96 (2017): n. pag.

Due to the increasing amount of thyroid disease in China, Chinese scientists decided to investigate the relationship between prevalence of thyroid disease and different urinary iodine concentrations in populations residing in mainland

China. They included forty-three articles in this systematic review and meta-analysis. They found the prevalence of thyroid nodules was 22.3%, 25.4% and 6.8% for low-iodine group, medium-iodine group, and high-iodine group, respectively. Thus, the prevalence of thyroid nodules in the populations with the highest iodine intake was significantly the lowest. Additionally, the authors indicated that the prevalence of most thyroid diseases is lowest for urinary iodine concentrations ranging from 100 to 299 µg/l.

Grussendorf M, Reiners C, Paschke R, Wegscheider K: **Reduction of thyroid nodule volume by levothyroxine and iodine alone and in combination: a randomized, placebo-controlled trial.** J Clin Endocrinol Metab 2011;96:2786-2795.

As the prevalence of thyroid nodules is high, up to 30% in Europe alone, other scientists conducted this prospective, double-blind, randomized, placebo-controlled trial to evaluate the effect of iodine and T4 supplementation on volume of thyroid nodules and thyroid. The study included 1024 euthyroid patients aged 18-64 years with one or more thyroid nodules. These patients were given iodine (150 µg potassium iodide), T4 (75 µg levothyroxine), iodine plus T4, or a placebo for 12 months. As it turned out, after the 1 year period, nodule volume reductions were -17.3% for the combined treatment group (T4+I), -7.3% for the T4 treatment group and -4.0% for the iodine treatment group compared to placebo. The combination of these two therapeutic measures was therefore most effective. As for thyroid volume reductions, they were -7.9%, -5.2%, -2.5% respectively. Hence, from the results of this study, we can conclude that even a relatively small dose of iodine may be effective in reducing thyroid nodules and in combination with T4 even more.

Knudsen, Nils et al. "**Comparative study of thyroid function and types of thyroid dysfunction in two areas in Denmark with slightly different iodine status.**" European journal of endocrinology 143 4 (2000): 485-91 .

Danish scientists wanted to compare the prevalence of thyroid dysfunctions in two regions in Denmark with slightly different iodine excretion. To this end, they selected 4649 participants aged between 18 and 65 years from the Civil Registration System in Denmark and collected blood samples from them, evaluated questionnaires and used ultrasonography. In Aalborg, the median iodine excretion was 53 µg/L, whereas in Copenhagen it was 68 µg/L. Not previously diagnosed hyperthyroidism in people over 40 was found in 1.3% in Aalborg vs 0.5% in Copenhagen. The same pattern was true for not previously diagnosed hypothyroidism. In Aalborg, the prevalence of this disorder was 0.6% compared to 0.2% in Copenhagen. The scientists concluded: "Significant differences in thyroid dysfunction were found between the regions with a minor difference in iodine excretion. The findings are in agreement with a higher prevalence of thyroid autonomy among the elderly in the most iodine-deficient region."

Hypothalamus $\xrightarrow{\text{TRH}}$ Pituitary $\xrightarrow{\text{TSH}}$ Thyroid $\xrightarrow{}$ T4
$\xrightarrow{}$ T3

At this point, it is worth mentioning what the regulation of thyroid hormone secretion looks like in a nutshell. This can be seen in part above. The hypothalamus secretes thyrotropin-releasing hormone (TRH). This hormone stimulates the anterior pituitary to synthesize and release thyrotropin (TSH). TSH stimulates the synthesis of thyroid hormones and also stimulates the growth of the thyroid gland. This is when the thyroid gland releases T4 and T3 into the blood, which results in the increase in metabolism. However, we also have negative feedback here. By acting on the pituitary, T4 and T3 inhibit the release of TSH. Likewise, by acting on the hypothalamus, these hormones inhibit the release of TRH. If that's understandable, let's move on to research into the relationship between iodine and various thyroid diseases. We will see, among other things, that higher doses of iodine do not cause them, but rather protect against them.

Teng W, Shan Z, Teng X, et al. **Effect of iodine intake on thyroid diseases in China**. N Engl J Med 2006; 354: 2783–93.

In this study, researchers analyzed cohorts from three regions in China with different levels of iodine intake (median urinary iodine excretion), which they defined as mild deficiency (84 μg/L), more than adequate (243 μg/L) and excessive (651 μg/L). Over three thousand participants were followed for five years. The cumulative incidence of overt hypothyroidism for the mildly iodine deficient group, more than adequate iodine intake and with excessive iodine intake was 0.2%, 0.5% and 0.3% respectively. Overt hypothyroidism is when TSH levels are elevated and T4 levels lowered. Hypothyroidism can be accompanied by symptoms such as cold hands and feet, constipation, depression, hypertension, fatigue, hair loss, weight gain or menstrual problems. In this case, the excessive amount of iodine was not associated with a higher cumulative incidence of this ailment. Regarding subclinical hypothyroidism, cumulative incidence was 0.2%, 2.6% and 2.9%, respectively. Subclinical hypothyroidism is when TSH levels are elevated at normal T4 levels. Since the attempt to diagnose certain symptoms specific for this disorder in some patients has failed, the diagnosis can only be made on the basis of laboratory tests. Experienced Dr David Brownstein stated that elevated TSH levels with normal T4 and T3 levels and the absence of clinical symptoms should not be identified as hypothyroidism. Later in this book, I'll also mention why starting iodine supplementation usually leads to elevated TSH levels, which is NIS-related and normal. Coming back to the study above, the cumulative incidence of overt hyperthyroidism was 1.4%, 0.9% and 0.8%, respectively. A higher iodine intake was therefore not associated with a higher amount of hyperthyroidism, quite the contrary. Cumulative incidence of Graves' disease was very similar in all regions. For autoimmune thyroiditis, the incidence was 0.2%, 1%, and 1.3%, respectively. The next studies I will present will be about thyroiditis and whether it is definitely caused by excessive iodine consumption. The last thing I will mention and have been monitored by researchers is the nodular goiter. Cumulative incidence of this disorder was 5%, 2.4% and 0.8% respectively. This result was therefore similar to those presented in earlier studies.

Okerlund MD. 1979. **The clinical utility of fluorescent scanning of the thyroid**. In: "Medical Applications of fluorescent excitation analysis". Kaufman L, Price D.C. edt., CRC Press Inc. (Florida) pp 149–160.

Dr. Okerlund measured the amount of iodine in the thyroid gland using X-ray fluorescence scanning. He found that the mean value of iodine per thyroid in the US population was 10 mg. In contrast, in the 56 patients suffering from autoimmune thyroiditis he scanned, the mean thyroid iodine value was only 4.8 mg. Furthermore, in 13 patients with autoimmune thyroiditis and hypothyroidism, the mean value was 2.3 mg per thyroid. If it was iodine that caused autoimmune thyroiditis, one would expect more of this element in the affected thyroid glands. Meanwhile, this study showed that there is 2 to 4 times less of it.

DeGroot, L.J., Thompson, J.E., & Dunn, A.D. (1965) Endocrinology 76, 632-639

In vitro studies with purified fractions of calf thyroid glands conducted by De Groot, et al showed that potassium iodide in concentrations of 10 μM has a protective effect (acts against oxidative damage) on TPO. TPO is a key enzyme involved in thyroid hormone synthesis. With an oxidized TPO, because of the absence of iodine, an autoimmune reaction occurs, damage to the apical membrane of the thyroid cells and, consequently, clinical symptoms of Hashimoto's thyroiditis. In order to achieve the mentioned concentration, which has TPO-protective properties, a person would have to ingest about 54 mg of iodide per day.

Data from Japan also indicated that the incidence of autoimmune thyroiditis is relatively low there. Average iodine consumption, in turn, is measured in this country in mg, not in μg. Milligram doses are also considered by the aforementioned Dr. Brownstein to be appropriate in the treatment of autoimmune thyroid diseases. From his practice and experience, they usually amount to 6 to 50 mg per day.

Although iodine does not appear to cause autoimmune thyroiditis in humans, some in vitro studies have shown that iodine can inhibit normal human thyroid cell proliferation. Such studies immediately frighten many, both ordinary readers and doctors. They are often the cause of the widespread fear of iodine. However, to obtain such an effect, iodine must be in mM concentration. This means that you would have to ingest iodine in gram amounts (many, even over 100 grams). Nobody mentally healthy recommends such amounts of iodine.

Wartofsky L, Ransil BJ, and Ingbar SH. **"Inhibition by iodine of the release of thyroxine from the thyroid glands of patients with thyrotoxicosis."** J Clin Invest, 1970; 49:78-86.

Doses similar to those used by Dr. Brownstein already proved to be beneficial in thyrotoxic patients fifty years ago. Wartofsky, et al administered five drops of lugol's solution three times a day (90 mg iodine/iodide per day) for 6-7 days to them. They reported: "For these reasons we would conclude that a decrease in the fractional rate of T4 release is at least the major reason that iodine acutely decreases T4 secretion, thereby decreasing serum T4 and ameliorating the clinical manifestations in patients with thyrotoxicosis". This means that iodine at a dose of 90 mg over several days induced a trend towards normalization of thyroid function. Therefore, this observation would indicate that hyperthyroidism should be treated with iodine, and not seen as caused by this element.

Sternthal, E, Lipworth, L, Stanley, B, Abreau, C, Fang, SL, Braverman, LE. **Suppression of thyroid radioiodine uptake by various doses of stable iodide.** N Engl J Med. 1980;303(19):1083–1088.

Sodium Iodide Ingested	Thyroid uptake of radioactive iodine (day 8)	Thyroid uptake of radioactive iodine (day 12)
10 mg	–	4%
15 mg	1.8%	1.9%
30 mg	1.3%	1.6%
50 mg	1.1%	1.2%
100 mg	0.6%	0.6%

As for radioactivity. Sternthal with fellow physicians studied the effects of various doses of sodium iodide on thyroid radioiodine uptake in euthyroid volunteers. Participants were given a single dose of 10, 30, 50, and 100 mg of iodide and then doses of 10, 15, 30, 50, or 100 mg daily for the next 12 days. The above table shows thyroid uptake of radioactive iodine on days 8 and 12 at particular of sodium iodide. Regarding the results of the study: "These data suggest that the thyroid uptake of radioactive iodine can be markedly suppressed by single-dose administration of 30 mg of stable iodide and that suppression can be maintained with daily doses of at least 15 mg. This study provides guidelines for stable iodide prophylaxis in the event of exposure to radioactive iodine. "

Abraham, G.E., Flechas, J.D., Hakala, J.C., **Orthoiodsupplementation: Iodine Sufficiency of the Whole Human Body**. The Original internist, 2002.

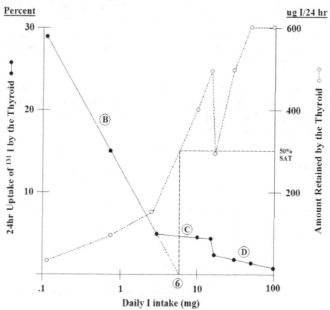

Fig. 2 - Percent 24hr uptake of radioiodide and computed uptake of I/24hr by the thyroid gland, following intake of increasing amount of I.

This graph shows the uptake of radioiodine/24h (percent) and computed uptake of iodine/24h by thyroid gland, following the intake of increasing amounts of iodine. As also shown in a previous study, with higher iodine intake the uptake of radioactive iodine decreases. At that time, there is also an increasing saturation of the thyroid with iodine. As we can see at a dose of about 6 mg serum inorganic iodide is in dynamic equilibrium (balance between reaction rate) with the exchangeable pool of inorganic iodide in the thyroid gland. The maximum amount that did not induce the autoregulatory mechanism of the thyroid gland was 14 mg. The doctor stated: "This amount may represent the upper limit of I required for sufficiency of the whole human body". After the dose of above about 15 mg of iodine the efficiency of the trapping mechanism further increases and reaches its maximum with a dose of 50 mg. This maximum daily thyroidal uptake was estimated at 0.6 mg/day.

CHAPTER 69:
CARDIOVASCULAR
HEALTH

In the past medicine, there has been a long tradition of using iodine for heart disease (atherosclerosis). Although it was not known exactly how iodine works in this disease, it seemed to be effective. The daily dose was as high as 500-700 mg of potassium iodide three times a day. This is 10,000 to 14,000 times the recommended daily dose of iodine. Nowadays, iodine has been forgotten in this regard, and I hope this short chapter will remind doctors and everyone else about its properties in cardiovascular health.

Cann, S. (2006). Hypothesis: **Dietary Iodine Intake in the Etiology of Cardiovascular Disease.** Journal of the American College of Nutrition, 25, 1 - 11.

Stephen A. Hoption Cann proposed the hypothesis that iodine deficiency can have deleterious effects on the cardiovascular system and therefore increasing the supply of this element would be beneficial. He pointed out that promoting salt restriction (which is some source of iodine in the population) to prevent hypertension and cardiovascular disease could be counterproductive. In the United States, the National Health Survey in the 1970s found that 1 in 40 people had iodine levels indicating moderate or greater deficiency. Twenty years later, 1 in 9 people were severely deficient in iodine. As many studies have shown and as I mentioned earlier, iodine deficiency is closely related to such ailments as hypothyroidism and hyperthyroidism. These diseases, in turn, are associated with a higher risk of heart disease. Although iodine itself has been used in the past as a treatment for cardiovascular disease and hypertension, we have very little modern studies that deal with this topic.

Zalawadiya, Sandip K. et al. "Abstract 16854: **Iodine Deficiency and Risk of Coronary Heart Disease Events Among Low Risk Healthy US Adults.**" Circulation 124 (2011): n. pag.

The authors of the above cross-sectional study wanted to evaluate the effect of iodine deficiency on primary risk of coronary heart disease events. To this end, they analyzed the health data of 10,037 adults who were free of cardiovascular disease and diabetes and participated in the National Health and Nutrition Examination Surveys. They then assessed the Framingham risk score (that estimates the 10-year cardiovascular risk of an individual) and their urine iodine levels. The mean Framingham risk score for those with higher urine iodine levels (over 100 µg/L) was 7.5 compared with 9.4 for those with the lowest levels (under 50 µg/L). Therefore, iodine deficiency was associated with coronary heart disease risk. This risk turned out to be independent of thyroid dysfunction and traditional cardiovascular risk factors.

Herter-Aeberli, Isabelle et al. "**Iodine Supplementation Decreases Hypercholesterolemia in Iodine-Deficient, Overweight Women: A Randomized Controlled Trial.**" The Journal of nutrition 145 9 (2015): 2067-75 .

The purpose of this randomized controlled intervention was to investigate the effect of iodine supplementation on serum TSH, plasma total and LDL cholesterol. The study included 163 iodine-deficient and overweight or obese Moroccan women who received 200 µg oral iodine or a placebo daily for 6 months. During this time, the median urinary iodine concentration increased from 38 µg/L to 77 µg/L. On the other hand, after 6 months, TSH was 33% lower in the iodine group than in the placebo group. Moreover, total cholesterol in subjects with elevated baseline cholesterol (over 5 mmol/L) was reduced by 11% after the supplementation. In the treated group, at 6 months, 21.5% of treated women remained hypercholesterolemic (from the initial 44.2%), whereas in the control group it was 34.8% (from the initial 36.8%). Also the prevalence of elevated LDL cholesterol in the iodine supplement group decreased from 50.6% to 35.4% compared with 47.4% to 44.9% in the control group (however, it was not a statistically significant reduction). The researchers concluded: "Our findings suggest that moderate to severe iodine deficiency in overweight women elevates serum TSH and produces a more atherogenic lipid profile and that iodine supplementation in this group reduces the prevalence of hypercholesterolemia. Thus, iodine prophylaxis may reduce cardiovascular disease risk in overweight adults."

CHAPTER 70:
DIABETES

Some studies have shown that iodine levels are inversely associated with the blood glucose levels. That is, the higher iodine levels are related to the decreased blood glucose levels. Likewise, it has been found that pregnant and lactating women in areas with significantly higher water iodine levels have a lower risk of hyperglycemia and it is an independent protective factor for this condition. This observation seems to be consistent with that of Dr. Jorge Flechas in his medical practice.

Flechas, J.D., **Orthoiodosupplementation in a primary care practice**. The Original Internist, 12(2):89-96, 2005.

Dr. Jorge Flechas discovered this link by chance while treating a 320-pound woman with insulin dependent diabetes. The woman received standard treatment, was given insulin and had to control glucose levels at home using a glucometer. Two weeks later, she returned to the office for a checkup of her insulin dependent diabetes. During the examination, it turned out that the woman also had fibrocystic breast disease. Therefore, the doctor recommended that she start iodine therapy in the amount of 50 mg per day. A week later the woman called the doctor asking for a reduction in insulin dose due to problems with hypoglycemia. She was told to drop her insulin levels and continue sugar monitoring. Four weeks later, the woman came for a medical appointment. The glucometer record indicated that the woman had average random blood sugar of 98, moreover, she gave up insulin three weeks earlier and did not take any medications to lower blood sugar during this time. She felt it was because of the iodine. Two years later, she still had "excellent glucose control" on 50 mg of iodine per day. Since then, Dr. Jorge Flechas, et al, also conducted a study on twelve people with diabetes. After supplementation of 50 to 100 mg of iodine per day, half of the patients could discontinue all diabetes-related medications as well as maintain hemoglobin A1C of less than 5.8 with the average random blood sugar of less than 100. The total amount of diabetes-related medications needed was reduced in all patients. In addition, also in type 1 diabetes, the doctor reported the effectiveness of iodine (50 mg/day) in reducing insulin required if C-peptide is measurable.

CHAPTER 71:
IMMUNITY

Iodine appears to be an important factor in our immunity. Studies have shown that the addition of iodine contributed to immunoglobulin G (IgG) synthesis in human lymphocytes. IgG is designed to bind to the pathogen and to destroy it. Another important function of this antibody is to neutralize the toxins produced by pathogenic bacteria. IGg contributes to a much faster response of the body to the infection. A significant decrease in the level of immunoglobulin G in the blood, due to a variety of reasons, increases the patient's susceptibility to bacterial infections. However, this is not the only role iodine plays in maintaining proper immunity. It has been shown that iodine deficiency is associated with decreased phagocytic activity of blood neutrophils and decreased bactericidal properties of the plasma. Neutrophils are the most numerous group of all leukocytes and constitute approximately 70% of white blood cells. When a pathogen enters the body or tissue damage occurs, neutrophils begin to phagocytize the pathogenic compounds. To phagocytize means to engulf or ingest foreign cells or particles. Then they are neutralized by neutrophils with the help of enzymes. Iodine deficiency is likely to contribute to the lack of this important activity. Although there are few studies into the relationship between iodine and the immune system, there are some that clearly indicate the existence of such a relationship.

Derscheid RJ, van Geelen A, Berkebile AR, Gallup JM, Hostetter SJ, et al. (2014) **Increased concentration of iodide in airway secretions is associated with reduced respiratory syncytial virus disease severity**. Am J Respir Cell Mol Biol 50: 389-397.

One of them examining the effect of iodine on immunity has been carried out on animals. Newborn lambs were given potassium iodide by intragastric gavage or were left untreated before intratracheal inoculation of respiratory syncytial virus. Sheep treated with potassium iodide had a 10-fold increase in airway surface liquid (ASL) concentration (which is important in mucociliary clearance and antimicrobial properties of the airway). Moreover, gross lung lesions, expiratory effort, IL-8 and pulmonary expression of an respiratory syncytial virus antigen was reduced in sheep treated with iodide compared to untreated sheep. In a similar experiment with 3-week-old lambs, administration of potassium iodide was associated with a reduction in gross lesions, a reduction in respiratory syncytial virus titers in bronchoalveolar lavage fluid, and a reduction in respiratory syncytial virus antigen expression. Overall, potassium iodide has been shown to be effective in reducing the severity of respiratory syncytial virus infections.

Additionally, several studies showed that Iodine-rich Tasco-Forage, an extract from the brown seaweed Ascophyllum nodosum, led to increased antioxidant activity as well as enhanced immune function in grazing animals.

Marani L, Venturi S. Iodio e immunità ritardata [**Iodine and delayed immunity**]. Minerva Med. 1986 May 7;77(19):805-9. Italian. PMID: 3714096.

Italian researchers Marani and Venturi found significant immune deficiencies in iodine-deficient children. Despite these present deficiencies and the low urinary iodine excretion levels, both T4, T3, and TSH were normal. Hence, they decided to establish a relationship between dietary iodine and immune response. 607 infants residing in an area of endemic goiter were included in the study. 215 of them received 2 mg of Lugol's solution per week (i.e. about 285 µg per day) for 8 months, while 392 received no iodine. The immune response was assessed by the skin test method. As it turned out, iodine supplementation restored in these children a normal immune response and the conclusion was: "The results appear to indicate that an adequate iodine intake is necessary for normal retarded immune response."

Fischer, Anthony J. et al. **"Enhancement of respiratory mucosal antiviral defenses by the oxidation of iodide."** American journal of respiratory cell and molecular biology 45 4 (2011): 874-81 .

The authors of the above publication presented a certain mechanism of iodine action leading to the enhancement of antiviral immunity. They showed that iodine delivered to respiratory epithelial cells supports the generation of strongly antimicrobial substances. The iodine addition resulted in a marked reduction of both adenovirus transduction and respiratory syncytial virus titer. Furthermore, they administered a single dose of 130 mg of oral potassium iodide to human subjects. This resulted not only in higher iodide concentrations but also in the accumulation of iodide in upper airway secretions. The study therefore showed that high doses of iodine at one time can lead to amelioration of respiratory viral infections and lower but regular doses would probably be an effective preventive ingredient.

Old medical textbooks for the treatment of infectious diseases recommended doses of potassium iodide as high as 4-6 grams per day. Such doses have been used in the treatment of sporotrichosis, entomophthoromycosis or erythema multiforme. For inflammatory dermatoses, for example, the dose was about 1 gram per day divided into three doses. As an expectorant, potassium iodide was administered in doses of 5-6 grams per day. Topical iodine was also used to treat syphilis and lupus vulgaris. More recent data, in turn, suggested that iodine may lead to inhibition of vacuolation toxin activity of Helicobacter pylori. Hence, it is another possible way by which iodine can also prevent gastric cancer.

Pelletier J, Tessema B, Westover J, Frank S, Brown S, Capriotti J. 2020. **In Vitro Efficacy of Povidone-Iodine Nasal And Oral Antiseptic Preparations Against Severe Acute Respiratory Syndrome-Coronavirus 2 (SARS-CoV-2) medRxiv.**

In this study, povidone iodine nasal antiseptic formulations and PVP-I oral rinse antiseptic formulations (concentrations between 1% and 5%) were examined for virucidal efficacy against the SARS-CoV-2. Regardless of the concentration, both nasal antiseptics and oral rinse antiseptics resulted in complete inactivation of SARS-CoV-2. For this to happen, only 60 seconds of exposure to the agent was enough.

These results are similar to those obtained by many other studies. Scientists demonstrated high bactericidal efficacy of iodine against Klebsiella pneumoniae and Streptococcus pneumoniae, as well as the rapid inactivation of SARS-CoV, MERS-CoV, influenza virus A (H1N1) and rotavirus after just 15 seconds of iodine exposure. In addition, which can be absolutely crucial, iodine does not make bacteria resistant like antibiotics do.

Brownstein, David G. et al. **"A Novel Approach to Treating COVID-19 Using Nutritional and Oxidative Therapies."** (2020).

Dr David Brownstein, Dr Richard Ng, et al, conducted an observational case series study on patients diagnosed with COVID-19. One hundred and seven of them who were either diagnosed as COVID-19 positive by PCR nasal swab testing or presumed to have COVID-19 due to symptomatology were included in the study. The most common symptoms of patients in the total cohort (n=107) were: fever (81%), shortness of breath (68%), symptoms including cough (69%), symptoms like diarrhea, loose stools, pain (27%). In the cohort of patients tested positive for COVID-19 (n = 27), these were 93%, 74%, 78%, and 33%, respectively. 99% of patients (n = 106) received oral treatment as the protocol of oral supplements, including vitamin A (100000 IU/day), vitamin D (50000 IU/day), vitamin C (1 gram/hour while awake until bowel tolerance), and iodine (25 mg/day in the form of Lugol's solution or tableted Lugol's solution). Additionally, 30% received intravenous hydrogen peroxide, 35% intravenous vitamin C (2.5 grams of sodium ascorbate), and 35% intramuscular ozone injections. Almost all people (85%) received a nebulized solution of normal saline and dilute hydrogen peroxide and (85%) nebulized iodine. Patients reported the first improvement after an average of 2.4 days, feeling mostly better after 4.4 days and feeling completely better after 6.9 days from the start of treatment. Only three people were hospitalized, two of whom were hospitalized before beginning the treatment. Overall, of all those treated, all recovered. In other words, there were no COVID-19 related deaths. Despite the fact that there was no control group, it can be concluded that the treatment results were very good. For example, at that time in the state of Michigan the case fatality rate was 9.0%. If this had been the case for this cohort at the time, at least a few people should have died. It is a pity that, despite the fact that more than two years have passed since this very promising publication, there are still no randomized controlled trials carried out and, more importantly, no effective treatment has been applied on a large scale.

Boretti, A., & Banik, B.K. (2021). **Potential Effects of Iodine Supplementation on Inflammatory Processes and Toxin Removal Following COVID-19 Vaccination.** Biological Trace Element Research, 200, 3941 - 3944.

We already know that iodine exhibits strong virucidal activities against SARS-CoV-2. Povidone-iodine has been shown to be able to inactivate the virus quickly. Furthermore, povidone-iodine mouthwash, gargle, and nasal spray have been shown to significantly reduce viral load in patients with COVID-19. Overall, iodine is also an extremely important substance in human immunity, and oral administration may be helpful for COVID-19 as well. The co-author of a previous study, Dr. David Brownstein, recommended 25-100 mg and more if ill of iodine per day. However, it seems that not only in this above, iodine plays a big role. Boretti and Banik suggested that iodine may be a possible agent to limit vaccine adverse events. As it turns out, iodine strongly increases the mRNA decay rate. Hence, although the toxicity of mRNA is marginally researched, scientists indicated iodine may prevent some of the damages caused by COVID-19 mRNA vaccines. Iodine is also known for its other detoxifying properties (for example, iodine binds to aluminum and mercury), which could also be important in the case of non-replicating COVID-19 viral vectors vaccines.

CHAPTER 72: PREGNANCY, NEURODEVELOPME NT

This chapter is extremely important, especially for women who are planning to have a child and get pregnant. The National Health and Nutrition Examination Survey (NHANES) 2005-2010 showed that the median urinary iodine concentrations of pregnant women indicate iodine insufficiency. A study from Europe found that women in two-thirds of European countries were iodine deficient during pregnancy. Overall, the median of iodine intake of pregnant women was shown to be insufficient in 75% of the studies that were analyzed. This, of course, is not good, even very bad, and has serious consequences. These consequences can affect both the pregnant woman and her child and involve stillbirth, miscarriage, placenta previa, preeclampsia, neonatal hypothyroidism, hypothyroxinemia, intellectual development, IQ and ADHD. I hope that the studies I mentioned will convince every future mother of the importance of taking care of iodine intake and that of every future father of the importance of caring for his woman. We'll start with a few animal studies.

Animal studies

Li, J.Q., Wang, X., Yan, Y., Wang, K., Qin, D., Xin, Z., and Wei, J. 1985. **The effects of severely iodine deficient diet derived from an endemic area on fetal brain development in the rat**. Observations in the first generation. Neuropathol. and Appl.

Neurobiol. 12:261-270.

The above study was conducted on rats fed on a severely iodine deficient diet (iodine content 4.5 µg/100 g). The diet was similar to that of the residents of Jixian village in China, who were severely deficient in iodine and had an 11% prevalence of endemic cretinism. It consisted mostly of crops like maize and wheat, vegetables, and water low in iodine. After 4 months of such a diet, in the intervention group, the thyroid and brain were tested in the adult and their fetuses. Then, the results of this group were compared with the results of the control group (diet with iodine content 54.7 µg/100 g). Scientists found marked goiters and reduced serum T4 in the intervention group. Furthermore, a higher uptake of 125I (radioisotope of iodine) by the thyroid and reduction in brain weight (combined with mean neuron size reduction) was also noted. Overall, iodine deficiency had a detrimental effect on rat fetuses.

Mano, M. T. et al. "Fetal brain development in response to iodine deficiency in a primate model (Callithrix jacchus jacchus)." *Journal of the Neurological Sciences* 79 (1987): 287-300.

Other researchers investigated the effects of dietary iodine deficiency on fetal brain development in marmoset (Callithrix jacchus jacchus). These animals were fed a low-iodine diet of maize, peas, meat meal, Torula yeast, maize oil and added vitamins, minerals and amino acids for 6 months before mating. Later, one group additionally received an iodine supplement. In iodine deficient fetuses at birth, reduced plasma T4 levels, increased plasma TSH levels, increased thyroid weight (enlarged thyroid gland) and reduced thyroid iodine content were observed. There was a significant reduction in the weight of the fetal brain, especially the cerebellum. Histology of the brain revealed morphological changes in the cerebellum and a significant reduction in brain cell number there. The newborn deficient marmosets showed also some sparsity of hair growth. All these unfavorable changes related to the second pregnancy more than the first one, suggesting greater iodine deficiency then.

Potter BJ, Mano MJ, Belling GB, McIntosh GH, Hua C, CraggBGet al. **Retarded foetal brain development resulting from severe dietary iodine deficiency in sheep.**Neuropathol-Appl-Neurobiol 1982; 8: 303–313.

A similar study was performed by B. J. Potter, et al, on sheep in which severe iodine deficiency was produced through a diet low in iodine (sheep were fed crushed maize and pelleted pea pollard). In iodine-deficient sheep, researchers noticed both fetal hypothyroidism and thyroid hyperplasia (thyroid enlargement) from 70 days gestation. There was a significant reduction in body and brain weight as well as brain DNA. The brain retardation was present and the deformation of the skull. The absence of wool growth and delayed skeletal maturation near parturition was also characteristic. The cerebellum changes were similar to those reported in the previous study. The same scientist also showed in his earlier study that single intramuscular injection of iodized oil given to the mother deficient in iodine at 100 days gestation leads to partial restoration of the lambs' both brain and body weight as well as maternal and fetal plasma T4 values.

Human studies

Kemp WN. **IODINE DEFICIENCY IN RELATION TO THE STILLBIRTH PROBLEM.** Can Med Assoc J. 1939 Oct;41(4):356-61. PMID: 20321492; PMCID: PMC537512.

As early as 1939, Dr. W. N. Kemp published a study suggesting a direct relationship between iodine deficiency during pregnancy and stillbirths. He found that the administration of iodine to pregnant women almost completely prevented stillbirths in Vancouver over the course of several years. The work of Lomer and others early investigators would indicate that iodine deficiency may cause abortion in some instances. In addition, the medical experience of Lomer, Lehmann and others in administering very high doses of potassium iodide to pregnant women suggested that women were more tolerant of this element during pregnancy without untoward results.

Dillon, J.C., & Milliez, J. (2000). **Reproductive failure in women living in iodine deficient areas of West Africa.** BJOG: An International Journal of Obstetrics & Gynaecology, 107.

Dillon and Millez investigated the association between iodine status and reproductive failure in a population of West African (iodine deficient areas of Senegal) women. 4908 women, including 1544 adolescents and 462 pregnant women, were examined in terms of the size of the thyroid gland and urinary iodine excretion. They found that repeated miscarriages and stillbirth was significantly associated with low iodine status. The risk increased with the severity of iodine deficiency and was more than three times higher compared to the group with iodine sufficiency.

Pharoah, P.O., & Connolly, K.J. (1987). **A Controlled Trial of Iodinated Oil for the Prevention of Endemic Cretinism: A Long-Term Follow-Up.** International Journal of Epidemiology, 16, 68-73.

In the mid-1960s, in Papua New Guinea, a double blind controlled trial was begun to examine the effectiveness of intramuscular iodinated oil as a prophylactic for endemic cretinism. Infants born between 1966 and 1972 were included into the study and followed up until 1982. There was a striking difference in the 15-year cumulative survival rate between the iodine group and the non-iodine group in favor of the iodine group. Moreover, the study showed that if the iodine was given before conception the nervous form of endemic cretinism was prevented. Children born to mothers given an iodine supplement performed significantly better, as shown by the measures of motor and intellectual function.

DeLong GR, Leslie PW, Wang SH, et al: **Effect on infant mortality of iodination of irrigation water in a severely iodine-deficient area of China.** Lancet 1997;350:771-773.

As Hotien county in Xinjiang province, China, was an area with widespread severe iodine deficiency and high infant mortality, researchers decided to investigate whether iodine replacement through iodination of the irrigation water would decrease this mortality. They added potassium iodate to irrigation water in certain areas of three townships (Tusala, Long Ru, and Bakechi). Hence, in women of child-bearing age the median urinary iodine concentration significantly increased from below 10 ug/L to 55 ug/L. Infant-mortality rates decreased in the treated areas of Long Ru from mean 58.2/1000 births to 28.7/1000 births, Tusala from 47.4/1000 births to 19.1/1000 births, and Bakechi from 106.2/1000 births to 57.3/1000 births. Additionally, similar results also applied to neonatal mortality. Overall, iodine replacement has probably been an important factor in the national decrease in infant mortality in China.

Cao, X. Y. et al. **"Timing of vulnerability of the brain to iodine deficiency in endemic cretinism."** The New England journal of medicine 331 26 (1994): 1739-44.

The authors of this publication systematically administered iodine to a group of 689 children from birth to three years of age and 295 women at each trimester of pregnancy. These participants lived in the aforementioned iodine-deficient area of the Xinjiang region of China. Researchers wanted to investigate the relationship between iodine and neural development in children. They found that the prevalence of moderate or severe neurologic abnormalities in infants whose mothers received iodine in the first or second trimester was 2% compared with 9% in infants whose mothers received iodine in the third trimester or after birth. The prevalence of microcephaly was 11% for iodine-treated children, whereas in iodine-untreated children was 27%. Furthermore, the developmental quotient at two years of age was 90 for iodine-treated children versus 75 for iodine-not treated children. Overall, up to the end of the second trimester iodine supplementation was the most effective. The results of this study therefore indicated that women who plan to become pregnant should ensure the adequate intake of iodine throughout pregnancy in order to ensure the child's proper neural development, among other things.

The use of iodized salt in Bangladesh, India, Nepal, and Sri Lanka also contributed to positive, though slightly smaller results compared to the previous study. Such an addition during pregnancy was related to increased weight for age and an increased mid-upper-arm circumference during infancy.

Businge, Charles Bitamazire et al. **"Insufficient iodine nutrition status and the risk of pre-eclampsia: a protocol for systematic review and meta-analysis."** BMJ Open 9 (2019): n. pag.

The results of this systematic review and meta-analysis published by scientists from South Africa also suggest an association between iodine deficiency and pre-eclampsia. Preeclampsia is a medical condition that occurs during pregnancy and is characterized by high blood pressure, protein in their urine, and, less frequently, headaches or blurred vision. After analyzing five different studies, these researchers concluded that the frequency of the occurrence of this ailment may be related to the level of iodine. They found that the overall proportions of preeclampsia among women with urinary iodine concentration <150 μg/L and >150 μg/L in two cross-sectional studies were 203/214 and 67/247, respectively. Moreover, in two cohort studies the overall incidence of preeclampsia was 6/1411 and 3/2478, respectively, for the same iodine division as before. Thus, lower urinary iodine concentrations (<150 μg/L) were associated with a 2.85 times higher risk of pre-eclampsia (the result, however, was statistically insignificant at P=0.09).

Yang J, Liu Y, Liu H, Zheng H, Li X, Zhu L, et al. **Associations of maternal iodine status and thyroid function with adverse pregnancy outcomes in Henan Province of China**. J Trace Elem Med Biol. (2018) 47:104–10. doi: 10.1016/j.jtemb.2018.01.013

The authors of the above publication from 2018 investigated the effects of maternal iodine status and thyroid diseases on adverse pregnancy outcomes. Both urinary iodine concentration and thyroid function were measured in 2,347 participants of this prospective cohort study. As it turned out, pregnant women who had urinary iodine concentration between 150 and 249 μg/L had lower incidences of preeclampsia, placenta previa and fetal distress than women with concentrations below 50 μg/L. Moreover, pregnant women with urinary iodine concentration between 100 and 149 μg/L had lower risks of abnormal amniotic fluid and also fetal distress. The researchers found that in the case of clinical and subclinical hypothyroidism, the risk of preterm delivery increases by 4.4 times and 3 times, respectively. Additionally, hyperthyroidism was found to be significantly associated with miscarriages. The above disorders, as mentioned before, can be also closely related to iodine deficiency.

Kochupillai, N., and Pandav, C.S. 1987. **Neonatal chemical hypothyroidism in iodine-deficient environments. In The prevention and control of Iodine Deficiency Disorders**. B.S.

Hetzel, J.T. Dunn, and J.B. Stanbury, editors. Amsterdam: Elsevier publ. 85-93.

Kochupillai, Pandav, et al, investigated the relationship between neonatal chemical hypothyroidism and iodine deficiency in newborns. Blood samples were taken from the umbilical vein just after the birth of a newborn. In areas of Northern India which are severely deficient in iodine and more than 50% of the population have iodine levels below 25 μg per gram creatinine, the incidence of neonatal hypothyroidism was 75 to 115 per thousand births. By comparison, in Delhi, in a city where thyroid goiter prevalence is low and there is no cretinism, the incidence was 6 per 1,000 births. In the control area where goiter is absent, the prevalence of hypothyroidism was only 1 per 1000 births.

Other studies have also found a high incidence of neonatal hypothyroidism in areas affected by iodine deficiency. If iodine is not replenished in a timely manner, intellectual disability and physical development problems may occur in the child in the future. It is also believed that iodine deficiency before and during pregnancy may play a significant role in inducing maternal hypothyroxinemia. Hypothyroxinemia is defined as a normal maternal TSH concentration in conjunction with a low maternal free T4 concentration. There have been several studies already showing that iodine supplementation during pregnancy reduces the risk of maternal hypothyroxinemia. Hypothyroxinemia, unresolved by iodine administration, may be associated with the formation of goiter in both the mother and the fetus. Many observational studies have shown that in regions with severe iodine deficiency, the incidence of goiter during pregnancy is greater. Iodine deficiency is also associated with the thyroidal uptake of radioiodine which, interestingly, is highest in the earliest years of life and declines further over the course of life. Hence, in a child, iodine deficiency can contribute to increased uptake of the radioiodide resulting from nuclear radiation. To prevent this from happening, of course, the child should be given iodine.

Pretell EA, Palacios P, Tello L. **Iodine deficiency and the maternal/fetal relationship**. In: Stanbury JB, editor. Endemic

Goiter and Cretinism: Continuing Threats to World Health. Washington, DC: PAHO (1974). p. 143–55.

Prettel et al, conducted a study with the intention of examining the effects of iodine administration on endemic goiter and cretinism in three Andean villages with high incidences of goiter. More than 3,000 people were injected with iodized oil or placebo, 749 of whom were women of childbearing age. In women treated with iodine, mean daily urinary excretion during pregnancy was 543 µg, whereas in women who did not receive iodine it was only 25 µg. Initially, researchers found no differences between the cognitive outcomes of the offsprings of particular groups. However, this changed when children's iodine status was evaluated. Children in the iodine-sufficient group had significantly higher intelligence quotient (IQ) than children in the iodine-deficient group (85.6 vs 74.4).

Fierro-Benítez, Rodrigo et al. "**Effects on school children of prophylaxis of mothers with iodized oil in an area of iodine deficiency.**" Journal of Endocrinological Investigation 11 (1988): 327-335.

Other researchers wanted to examine the effects of iodine on intellectual and psychomotor performance and school performance in children from a rural impoverished and iodine deficient Andean whose mothers received injections of iodinated oil during the first trimester of pregnancy. Two villages (where the women got and did not get iodine) were followed for 20 years, and the neurophysiological effects on the offspring were monitored. Children whose mothers got iodine during pregnancy performed better on tests of psychomotor maturation. Furthermore, they performed even better when evaluated in terms of school drop-out rates, grades achieved and repeated, and in overall performance as judged by teacher notes.

Zimmermann, Michael B. et al. "**Iodine supplementation improves cognition in iodine-deficient schoolchildren in Albania: a randomized, controlled, double-blind study.**" The American journal of clinical nutrition 83 1 (2006): 108-14.

This randomized, controlled, double-blind study, in turn, examined the effect of administering iodine to children on their cognitive and motor performance. 310 children aged 10-12 from rural southeastern Albania with low iodine urinary concentrations were given 400 mg of iodine (as oral iodized oil) or a placebo. These children later had to solve several tests checking information processing, working memory, visual search, visual problem solving and fine motor skills. As it turned out, iodine administration significantly improved performance in rapid target marking, symbol search, rapid object naming, and Raven's Colored Progressive Matrices (used to measure general human intelligence and abstract reasoning).

Gordon, Rosie et al. "**Iodine supplementation improves cognition in mildly iodine-deficient children.**" The American journal of clinical nutrition 90 5 (2009): 1264-71 .

A similar study was conducted by scientists at the University of Otago in New Zealand who wanted to investigate whether supplementing mildly iodine-deficient children with iodine improves cognition. In this randomized, placebo-controlled, double-blind trial, 184 children aged 10-13 years were given either 150 µg of iodine or a placebo for 28 weeks. Iodine supplementation had a significant impact on the improvement of cognitive test scores for picture concepts and matrix reasoning. The authors concluded: "Iodine supplementation improved perceptual reasoning in mildly iodine-deficient children and suggests that mild iodine deficiency could prevent children from attaining their full intellectual potential."

Lombardi, Fabrizio Aghini et al. "**Mild iodine deficiency during fetal/neonatal life and neuropsychological impairment in Tuscany.**" Journal of Endocrinological Investigation 18 (1995): 57-62.

Italian researchers studied the neuropsychological performance of schoolchildren living in areas with present and past iodine deficiency in Tuscany. They tested neuropsychological performance in 107 children with a median urinary iodine excretion of 64 ug/L living in Borgo a Mozzano, an area of mild iodine deficiency as well as in 106 children with a median urinary iodine excretion of 142 ug/L living in Marina di Pisa, an iodine sufficient coastal village. Such tests were also carried out in 57 children living in the village of Vagli, of which 30 were born before iodine prophylaxis (32 µg/L) and 27 after starting iodine prophylaxis (109 µg/L). After analyzing the results, the authors came to two conclusions; first, even mild iodine deficiency can contribute to disturbing the rate of motor response to perceptive stimuli, also in the absence of general cognitive impairment, second, the effects of iodine deficiency during fetal/neonatal life may be present in later years whether the deficiency was corrected later or not.

Santiago-Fernández, Piedad et al. "**Intelligence quotient and iodine intake: a cross-sectional study in children.**" The Journal of clinical endocrinology and metabolism 89 8 (2004): 3851-7 .

A similar study to the previous one was carried out by Spanish scientists on 1221 school children from southern Spain in which urinary iodine excretion was measured. They found that intelligence quotient (IQ) was significantly higher in children with urinary iodine levels above 100 µg/l. On the other hand, children who had urinary iodine levels lower than 100 µg/L had a higher risk of having an IQ below 70. Based on these results, the researchers suggested a possibility of improving the IQ by ensuring adequate iodine intake in children (the sooner the better).

Bleichrodt, N., & Born, M.P. (1996). **A metaanalysis of research on iodine and its relationship to cognitive development.**

Bleichrodt and Born in a meta-analysis of 19 studies on neuromotor and cognitive functions in conditions of moderate to severe iodine deficiency concluded that iodine deficiency contributed to loss of 13.5 IQ points at the level of the global population.

Qian, Ming et al. "**The effects of iodine on intelligence in children: a meta-analysis of studies conducted in China.**" Asia Pacific journal of clinical nutrition 14 1 (2005): 32-42 .

A few years later, Chinese scientists published a meta-analysis with results similar to the previous of Bleichrodt and Born. They analyzed 37 studies (comparing children living in iodine sufficient and iodine deficient areas as well as those from iodine deficient areas born before and after the introduction of iodine supplementation) including 12,291 children. The analysis showed that in children exposed to severe iodine deficiency intelligence damage was profound and amounted to 12.5 IQ points less. Moreover, an adequate iodine supplementation for mothers before and during gestation contributed to an increase in their children's IQ by 8.7 points.

Iodine deficiency has also been linked to attention deficit hyperactivity disorder (ADHD). In several studies, low iodine intake (<200 µg/day) was associated with higher child ADHD symptom scores. Moreover, most children with ADHD are iodine deficient.

CHAPTER 73:
MENSTRUAL
PROBLEMS AND
INFERTILITY

As we already know, iodine deficiency may contribute to both hypothyroidism and hyperthyroidism. These ailments, in turn, are associated with menstrual disorders as well as reproductive failure, including infertility, pregnancy wastage, and failure of lactation.

Joshi, Jaladhi et al. **"Menstrual irregularities and lactation failure may precede thyroid dysfunction or goitre."** Journal of postgraduate medicine 39 3 (1993): 137-41 .

To such conclusions also came the authors of the above publication after analyzing the menstrual and reproductive history of 178 women and comparing the results with 49 healthy controls. They found that only 31.8% of hypothyroid and 35.3% of hyperthyroid women had a normal menstrual pattern compared to 87.8% of healthy controls. Furthermore, reproductive failure (infertility, pregnancy wastage, failure of lactation) affected 37.5% of hypothyroid and 36.5% of hyperthyroid cases versus 16.7% of healthy controls. Interestingly, in a significant proportion of women, menstrual abnormality or reproductive failure and lactation failure preceded the diagnosis of thyroid disease, which may indicate that the main cause of all of this mentioned above is one. This one cause may be iodine deficiency.

Anecdotal evidence

1. The woman tried to have a child for a long time. At the time of visiting the clinic, it turned out that she had a lot of fibroids in her uterus and would probably never have children. She started Neprinol therapy, but stopped after two months. She then took Lugol's solution for several months in the amount of a few drops, and less than a month before her next visit to the doctor, she started taking 50 mg of iodine/iodide in the form of tablets per day. At the visit, it turned out that her uterus is healthy and there are no traces of fibroids.

2. The woman had cysts on the ovaries as well as uterine fibroid. She took 150 mg of iodine a day and also smeared iodine on abdomen. The cysts on the ovaries began to shrink. In addition, the uterine fibroid was gone.

CHAPTER 74:
FIBROMYALGIA

I have already written that in the case of fibromyalgia, an ailment characterized by extensive musculoskeletal pain accompanied often by chronic fatigue and sleep disturbance, vitamin D may prove very beneficial. However, doctors from their medical experience have also found that iodine may be another substance helpful in treating this disorder and reducing unpleasant symptoms. Some also conducted a small study.

Abraham, G.E., Flechas, J.D., **The Effect of Daily Ingestion of 100 mg Iodine Combined with High Doses of Vitamins B2 and B3 (ATP Cofactors) in Five Subjects with Fibromyalgia**. The Original Internist, 2008.

Dr. Guy E. Abraham and Dr. Jorge D. Flechas conducted a study investigating the effects of iodine alone and in combination with vitamins B2 and B3 in five patients with fibromyalgia. Three of them had severe fibromyalgia and two had moderate fibromyalgia (FIQ score). In the first phase of treatment, patients took 50 mg of iodine (Lodoral® tablet) twice a day for six weeks, in the second phase, in addition to 100 mg of iodine/day, the patients also took 200 mg of vitamin B2 and 1000 mg of vitamin B3 per day for the next six weeks. The Ghent score for severity of FBD decreased significantly after 12 weeks from the initial mean values SD of 14.6 to 5.4. The mean pressure threshold of tender points (kg/cm2) increased from an initial 51 to 63 after the first phase and 72 after the second phase. This can be seen in more detail in the table below.

	Pre-Intervention	Post-Phase I	Post-Phase II	p - Value
Fibromyalgia Impact Questionnaire (FIQ)	71	70	65	
Zung Depression Score	64	62	56	0.08
Pressure Threshold	51	63	72	0.07
Ghent's Score	14.6		5.4	0.02

Despite the fact that the emerging trends were promising, due to the small number of participants, they did not reach statistical significance. However, one patient responded remarkably well to the treatment. In the table below, I showed that response to intervention.

	Pre-Intervention	Post-Phase I	Post-Phase II
Fibromyalgia Impact Questionnaire (FIQ)	81	61	42
Zung Depression Score	75	64	55
Pressure Threshold	53	76	119
Ghent's Score	13		3

Importantly, the researchers did not observe any side effects in patients using both iodine alone and a combination of iodine with B vitamins. No statistically significant changes were also observed for urinalysis, blood chemistry, hematology, and body composition. These values remained within the normal ranges. There was also no significant change in mean thyroid volumes. However, there was a significant increase in TSH above baseline. In addition, there was a decrease of all thyroid hormones (total T4, total T3, free T4, and free T3) during the first phase, but the levels of these hormones returned to their baseline levels during the second phase.

CHAPTER 75: PCOS

Studies have shown that iodine deficiency negatively affects folliculogenesis in the maturation of the ovarian follicle, which in turn may lead to the development of polycystic ovary syndrome (PCOS). Abnormalities of early folliculogenesis have been significantly linked to increased Anti-Müllerian hormone concentrations (which is significantly higher in women with PCOS). Iodine, then, again turned out to be essential, in this case, for the proper functioning of the ovaries. Nonetheless, the link between PCOS and iodine has also been suggested indirectly by studies such as the one below.

Du, D., & Li, X. (2013). **The relationship between thyroiditis and polycystic ovary syndrome: a meta-analysis**. International journal of clinical and experimental medicine, 6 10, 880-9 .

As we already know from the section on thyroid, iodine deficiency is probably significantly associated with autoimmune thyroiditis (AIT). In turn, several studies have reported the link between AIT and PCOS. Hence, Du and Li decided to analyze six studies involving 726 PCOS patients and 879 controls to investigate this relationship closer. They found that the incidence of AIT in women with PCOS was 4.81 times greater than in the control groups. Moreover, two studies also reported the prevalence of goiter in people with PCOS. This prevalence in women with PCOS was 3.36 times higher than in the controls. Undeniably, the presence of goiter is also associated with iodine deficiency, which I have already proven on the basis of several publications.

Flechas, J.D., **Orthoiodosupplementation in a primary care practice**. The Original Internist, 12(2):89-96, 2005.

Dr. Flechas reported that he had five patients with polycystic ovarian syndrome at the time of writing the above article. These patients were treated with 50 mg of iodine per day. This therapy contributed to the disappearance of cysts and stabilization of periods. Moreover, type 2 diabetes mellitus was brought under control.

CHAPTER 76:
BROMINE AND
FLUORIDE

Brownstein, D.G. (2005). **Clinical Experience with Inorganic, Non-radioactive Iodine/Iodide.**

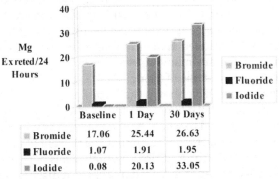

	Baseline	1 Day	30 Days
Bromide	17.06	25.44	26.63
Fluoride	1.07	1.91	1.95
Iodide	0.08	20.13	33.05

Dr. David Brownstein in his office conducted a study on eight randomized patients to evaluate their iodine levels as well as the amount of bromine and fluoride excreted in the urine. First, the excretion of these three elements in the urine was measured before the intervention. It is worth mentioning that no patient had been treated with iodine before. Then, these eight people took 50 mg of iodine/iodide in tablet form (Iodoral®) for 30 days. The averaged results of the study are presented above. As can be seen, iodine excretion increased during the 30 days of supplementation from 40.2% on the first day to 66.15% on the 30th day. This means that the body became more saturated with iodine and therefore excreted more iodine in the urine. Importantly, the body also got rid of more harmful halogens such as bromine and fluorine. On day 30, after iodine supplementation, the body excreted 56% more bromine and 82% more fluoride than before the supplementation. In a moment I will present why it is so crucial for health.

Bromine

Bromine along with chloride, fluoride, astatine and just our iodine belongs to the group of halogens. One thing that makes bromine harmful to our health is that it competes for the same receptors as iodine. Of course, in order for us to function at all, the thyroid gland must produce hormones for which iodine is essential. When our levels of bromine in the body are high, this element competes with iodine and the thyroid gland can no longer produce adequate amounts of thyroid hormones. Moreover, we know that the whole body needs iodine. Again, high levels of bromine compete with iodine and thus disrupt the work of many organs, which can eventually lead to disease. It should also be added that bromine itself has a toxic effect on tissues. There are many ailments scientists have linked to bromine. These are some of them:

- Animal studies have shown that bromine ingestion may contribute to both hypothyroidism and goiter. This is probably related to what I have already mentioned, that bromine displaces iodine, so that the thyroid gland cannot function properly. Additionally, high levels of bromine have been linked to autoimmune thyroid diseases such as Hashimoto's disease and Graves' disease.
- Scientists found significantly higher levels of bromine in cancerous thyroid tissue than in normal thyroid tissue, which may indicate the carcinogenic properties of bromine. A similar discovery was made in breast cancer, women with this type of cancer had significantly elevated levels of bromine. In addition, this element has also been linked to prostate and ovarian cancer.
- Bromine poisoning can cause delusions, hallucinations, psychosomatic delay, dementia, lethargy, cognitive impairment, schizophrenia and even suicidal thoughts.
- Bromine toxicity may also manifest itself in nodular acne, dryness and itching of the skin.

- Abdominal cramps and bloating may appear.
- Hearing impairment and even permanent deafness may also occur in the case of elevated bromine.

Unfortunately, humans are highly exposed to bromine and in most cases it cannot be prevented. Bromine is found in everything that surrounds us on a daily basis. Here is a list where we can find it:
- One of the greatest sources of bromine in the US population is bread. Potassium bromate is used extensively in baking to make the dough more elastic and of higher quality.
- Bromine is found in some fertilizers, so people also consume it with vegetables and fruits.
- Bromine has also been found in water.
- Bromine can be found in personal care products, including cosmetics (creams, shampoos, etc), hair dyes, permanent waves and fragrances.
- Bromine is found in cars (armrest, seats, upholstery).

If we are deficient in iodine, daily bromine exposure will be even more detrimental to us. Therefore, it is also one of the reasons why most people living in our toxic environment should increase their iodine intake.

Fluoride

Fluoride is another element in the family of halogens. Iodine, in turn, can greatly help us remove it from our body. This is crucial because fluoride is a poison to our body that contributes to many ailments later on. Here are some of them:
- Fluoride disturbs iodine uptake by the thyroid gland. Animal studies have shown that exposure to fluoride leads to goiter in iodine deficiency. Similarly, in humans, high fluoride intake in water was associated with a higher incidence of thyroid goiter.
- Fluoride has a negative effect on teeth and bones, contributing to dental fluorosis and fractures.
- Fluoride has been linked to many types of cancer, including breast cancer.
- Excess fluoride leads to lower intelligence, brain disorders,

and neurodegenerative diseases such as Azheimer's disease.
- Fluoride can lead to infertility in women.
- Fluoride poisoning can cause abdominal pain, nausea, vomiting and diarrhea.

Fluoride, like bromine, is ubiquitous in our lives. It is even in the water. In the past, water started to be fluoridated to prevent tooth decay. However, many scientists opposed this idea as not scientifically substantiated. Many observational studies have also shown that water fluoridation is ineffective in caries prevention. Even so, in many regions of the world, people still get fluoride from fluoridated water. Actually, it is not the only source of fluoride. Fluoride is found, for example, in many medications, including antibiotics, antidepressants, painkillers, and cholesterol-lowering drugs. This element can also be found in processed foods and beverages (which were made with the use of fluoridated water), tea or some food (made with fertilizers containing fluoride) such as rape products, cocoa powder and dried fruit. Fortunately, iodine in the right amount can significantly protect us from fluoride from the things mentioned above.

CHAPTER 77:
SAFETY OF IODINE

Iodism

Rarely, when the iodine dose is too high a person may experience iodism. The characteristic symptoms of this condition include: unpleasant metallic taste, coryza, increased salivation, sneezing and headache in the area of frontal sinuses. There may also be acne-like skin lesions. When symptoms of iodism appear, it is recommended to either reduce the dose of iodine or stop taking iodine. These symptoms should then disappear within a few days to three weeks. However, as already mentioned, the occurrence of iodism is rare. Dr. Guy Abrahem, el al, reported that in over 150 patients who supplemented with 12.5 mg of iodine per day, no side effects including any iodism were noted. In addition, practice has shown that the symptoms of iodism can be minimized by the use of certain substances. I will mention these substances soon.

Iodine allergy

The radioactive iodine used in various medical procedures is not the one found in e.g. Lugol's solution as iodine/iodide. Hence, people allergic to radioactive iodine are not necessarily allergic to the above-mentioned iodine. Likewise, those who are allergic to shellfish have concerns about iodine supplementation. However, most people allergic to shellfish can take iodine. It is not iodine that is causing the allergic reaction here. On the other hand, if a person is allergic to iodized salt, he or she is probably also allergic to iodine. Dr. David Brownstein claimed that in his twenty years of medical practice, he saw only three people who were allergic to inorganic and non-radioactive iodine, such as

Lugol's solution and Lugol's tablets. Furthermore, some patients can overcome the allergy using e.g. Nambudripad's Allergy Elimination Techniques (NAET).

Thyroid disorders

Many people worry that iodine supplementation can induce hypothyroidism, goiter, hyperthyroidism or cause autoimmune thyroid disease. Although I've already written a bit about this in the thyroid section, there are a few more things to mention. First, I need to describe some iodine-related mechanism that will explain many of the things that were discussed earlier in the book. Attentive readers have certainly noticed that many scientists reported significantly elevated TSH after starting iodine supplementation. I have previously written that TSH stimulates the thyroid gland to produce hormones. However, TSH also has another key function in the body. Namely, TSH also stimulates the body to produce sodium/iodide symporters (NIS), which allows iodine to enter the cell. If the subject is iodine deficient, his body requires a small amount of NIS so that the small amount of iodine consumed on a daily basis can also be transported into the cell. If, on the other hand, the patient starts supplementing with iodine, the body needs more NIS and therefore TSH increases significantly. It is a natural and appropriate reaction of the body. Experienced doctors say that an increase in TSH alone without any clinical symptoms and abnormal changes in T4 and T3 levels is not indicative of hypothyroidism. A transient decrease in T4 and T3 may appear, but it lasts up to several dozen hours. Increased TSH levels usually last up to six months after starting supplementation. Real cases of hypothyroidism or goiter induced by iodine administration, doctors report, are very rare. Dr. David Brownstein, et al, claim ed from experience with thousands of patients that iodine-induced hypothyroidism affects less than 0.1%. A similar statistic applies to hyperthyroidism, doctors report. However, if a patient has an autonomously functioning nodule on the thyroid gland, it may be associated with the development of hyperthyroidism. Then the patient has to avoid iodine from supplements and food and the nodule has to be surgically removed. In the case of autoimmune thyroid disease. I have mentioned several studies in the thyroid chapter suggesting that autoimmune thyroid disease is caused by an iodine deficiency rather than an iodine excess. Autoimmune diseases of the thyroid gland are also treated with iodine by many physicians who do not report the development of the disease in other iodine treated patients.

Detox

A few pages earlier, I described a study showing that iodine is able to significantly increase the excretion of bromine and fluoride from the body. This halogens excretion, for about 1 in 20 people, is associated with some symptoms like fatigue, brain fog, muscle ache or fever. These symptoms can be minimized or completely eliminated if supplementation is approached in an appropriate way. About this in a moment.

Abraham, Guy E.. **"The Safe and Effective Implementation of Orthoiodosupplementation In Medical Practice."** (2015).

To conclude this section, I will quote the respected Dr. Guy Abraham: "Of all the elements known so far to be essential for health, iodine is the most misunderstood and the most feared. Yet, it is by far the safest of all the trace elements known to be essential for human health. It is the only trace element that can be ingested safely in amounts up to 100,000 times the RDA. For example, potassium iodide has been prescribed safely to pulmonary patients in daily amounts of up to 6.0 gm/day, in large groups of such patients for several years. It is important, however, to emphasize that this safety record only applies to inorganic, non-radioiodides. Unfortunately, the severe side effects of iodine-containing drugs have been attributed to inorganic iodine/iodide, even though published studies clearly demonstrate that it is the whole organic molecule that is cytotoxic, not the iodine covalently bound to this molecule."

CHAPTER 78: REQUIREMENTS AND DEFICIENCY

In general, every cell in the body utilizes iodine. The thyroid gland contains the most iodine of all organs. However, other parts of the body also contain significant amounts of this element. These body parts include, for example, the breasts, ovaries, salivary glands, brain, gastric mucosa, and eyes. It has been estimated that the thyroid gland itself requires about 6 mg of iodine per day, and the (female) breasts about 5 mg of iodine per day. Totally, the human body may contain about 1.5-2 grams of iodine at sufficiency. This has been calculated on the basis of loading test, retention of iodine by subjects on 50 mg/day for three months. Fat tissue has been estimated to contain 700 mg of iodine and striated tissue 650 mg of iodine. For example, the thyroid gland can hold a maximum of about 50 mg of iodine. Consequently, the common belief that the thyroid gland contains 70% of the body's iodine and that the whole body contains only 15-20 mg of iodine is simply not true. That is also why iodine, as it affects all organs, has such a versatile therapeutic application. And it is not limited to the one mentioned by me. The effect of iodine has also been demonstrated in the case of: eczema, psoriasis, dry skin, allergy, feeling cold, blood pressure, cardiac arrhythmias, depression, ADHD, hair loss, gum pain, scarring, brain fog, fatigue, libido, vaginal infections, fertility (e.g. by lubricating the testicles with iodine diluted in oil), problems with vision, hearing loss, hemorrhoids and headaches.

On the other hand, iodine deficiency can contribute to the ailments mentioned above as well as those mentioned earlier.

This deficiency is very common. Between 1971-1974 and 1988-1994 only, the National Health and Nutrition Examination Surveys (NHANES) showed a significant decrease in urinary iodine levels by more than 50%. The average thyroid gland contains 10-20 mg of iodine, although as I just mentioned, it could be as much as 50 mg. NHANES from 2005-2008 showed that 56.9% of pregnant women have lower urinary iodine concentrations than those recommended by the World Health Organization (WHO). Moreover, currently over 2.2 billion people live in iodine-deficient areas as estimated by standard measurements of urinary iodine concentrations. Dr. David Brownstein et al, in turn, reported iodine deficiency in more than 96% of the patients out of 6,000 tested. They used a different, more reliable method to test the whole-body iodine status - the 24-hours iodine loading test. This test is based on the fact that if the level of iodine in the body is sufficient then most (> 90%) of the 50 mg of iodine taken at the beginning of the test will be excreted in the urine within 24 hours. If, in turn, we are deficient, more iodine will be absorbed and less will be excreted in the urine. It has been assumed that the urinary excretion of less than 90% of the ingested iodine indicates some deficiency. It is worth doing 24-hours iodine loading test before treatment with iodine.

NOTE: Sometimes the result of such a test may turn out to be false when the functioning of the NIS is impaired. Then iodine is ingested and quickly excreted in the urine. In this case, doctors recommend iodine supplementation for three months and repeat the test.

CHAPTER 79: INITIATION OF IODINE THERAPY

Although iodine, as already mentioned, is an extremely safe substance, the initiation of therapy may be associated with some unpleasant symptoms, mainly related to the excretion of metals such as bromine or fluoride. It is worth being well prepared for this. Below I will present what this may look like based on the experience of many doctors in the field of iodine treatment.

1. Drinking plenty of water with unrefined salt. Water is the basis for any body detoxification. It is also good if it was of good quality, above all clean. Salt has long been used to remove bromine from the body. Chloride, as we know, is in one family of halogens along with bromine. Therefore it is perfect for detoxifying this element. It is recommended to ingest at least one teaspoon of unrefined salt with water, and to salt the meals as well. Such therapy can be started a few days (or more) before iodine intake is started.

2. Ensuring an adequate supply of supporting substances. These substances include vitamin C in a dose of 3-9 grams per day (e.g. divided into 3 grams three times a day), magnesium in the amount of 300-500 mg per day (e.g. in the form of magnesium citrate), selenium in the amount of 100-200 mg per day and B vitamins. It should also be remembered about a diet rich in nutrients. Later, this diet can replace additional supplementation.

3. Iodine supplementation. Experienced doctors say doses of 12.5-50 mg of iodine per day are appropriate for most people. In the case of serious diseases such as, for example, breast cancer,

it may be more. Iodine is recommended in the form of Lugol's solution or in the form of tablets (e.g. Iodoral®), which contain both iodine and potassium iodide. This is because different parts of the body prefer different forms of iodine, the thyroid gland and skin prefers iodide, whereas the breast and prostate gland prefer iodine. Iodine in the form of Lugol's solution can be taken with e.g. fatty milk, cream or coconut milk to reduce the risk of irritation of the membranes. Some also recommend taking 48 hour breaks from iodine supplementation to give the kidneys a bit of rest during detoxification. In this case, iodine is supplemented for, for example, 5 days and a break is taken for 2 days.

CHAPTER 80:
THE OPTIMAL
DAILY DOSE

Back in the 1960s, one slice of bread contained as much iodine as today is the RDA for iodine for an entire day. From the bakery products alone, it was estimated that the average iodine intake had been 726 μg per day. Back then, one in twenty women got breast cancer. Nowadays, when iodine is replaced by bromine, statistics already speak of one in eight women. On the other hand, we have Japan, where one in thirty-eight women will be diagnosed with breast cancer. In the past, this prevalence was even lower. At the very beginning, I mentioned a study in which scientists estimated the daily iodine intake of Japanese people at 1 to 3 mg per day, i.e. 6.7-20 times the current RDA. However, it is not the only publication that addressed this issue. Earlier estimates reported an average iodine intake by Japanese people of about 5.3 mg of iodine per day. Additionally, it is worth noting that the range was between 1.8 and 13.7 mg of iodine per day. This means that there were some who consumed 1.8 mg of iodine a day (12x RDA), but also those who consumed 13.7 mg of iodine a day (91x RDA), mostly from seaweed. And this exact dose (i.e. about 13 mg/day) was considered by one of the most respected doctors in the field of iodine, Dr. Guy Abraham, as the one necessary to maintain iodine sufficiency. Although, as already mentioned, people with diseases related to the thyroid gland, breast, prostate, ovaries, uterus or skin may require more.

CONCLUSIONS

This is the right moment for a few conclusions from the book you have read to my delight. I wanted this book to be a little bit different from the others on similar topics. I wanted this book to be largely based on scientific studies and, to some extent, on the medical experience of doctors. The purpose of this was for the reader to see the broader picture. Usually, scientific studies indicate some preventive/therapeutic properties of a specific substance, while medical practice shows that, often at higher doses, this substance is extremely effective in treatment. I wanted to show these two sides. Unfortunately, at the moment there is a lack of large studies using doses that are/were successfully used by some doctors in their practice. Therefore, I have presented these two types of evidence. Another thing that, in turn, I did not want to do was waffle and waste the reader's time on unnecessary stories, as is the habit of many other authors. The book was to be dense in information and studies that are the best source of this information. Therefore, unlike other books, I have provided more details from these studies, not only "substance X was beneficial here". I hope this has helped better understand these three substances, how they work in our body, how safe they are, and what results we can expect from using them.

As for the results, I have proved hopefully they are very often extremely beneficial. I have shown that with the help of these three substances, we can significantly reduce the risk of developing many modern diseases that plague society and contribute to a huge number of deaths. I also proved that if the dose is high enough, it is possible to significantly reduce the symptoms and even completely cure the disease. The question of dose is particularly relevant here. To achieve the above, the dose must be appropriate, i.e. higher compared to the doses currently used. This applies to both prevention and treatment. Generalizing, as a society, we should consume higher amounts of both vitamin D, vitamin C and iodine to protect ourselves from many diseases, and in the event of illness, patients should be treated with these substances in appropriate amounts for the best results. This has been demonstrated by many scientific studies. Unfortunately, it seems that hardly anyone reads them. What's more, many doctors also belong to this group. Therefore, the last thing left is my request to recommend this book to family, friends and the doctor so that this knowledge spreads and may someday save lives.

FROM THE TEAM

If you have any comments, observations from the supplementation, or anything else you would like to share with Dr. Alexandre Doumenach, please write to the e-mail address - *dralexandredoumenach@gmail.com*. All messages will be forwarded to the doctor by his team.

We also ask you on behalf of Dr. Doumenach for your honest review on Amazon. This simple gesture will not only be an appreciation for the doctor's work, but also valuable information about the book for many people. Thank you very much.

Made in the USA
Middletown, DE
09 August 2023

36410437R00159